The Children's Sports Injuries Handbook

All care has been taken to ensure the accuracy and correctness of
the information in this book but no responsibility is accepted
for any errors or omissions. Bay Books Pty Ltd disclaim liability
for any damage or injury suffered by any persons acting upon or
relying on this book or the information contained in it. If pain
or discomfort persist or if there is any uncertainty about the
nature of an injury you should see your doctor.

This book is copyright. Apart from any fair dealing for the
purpose of private study, research, criticism or review, as
permitted under the Copyright Act, no part may be reproduced by
any process without written permission. Inquiries should be
addressed to the publisher.

© Copyright text Peter Fitzgerald with Dr David Kennedy

Published by Bay Books Pty Ltd
61–69 Anzac Parade
Kensington NSW 2033

National Library of Australia card number and
ISBN 1 86256 297 0

Designed by Greg Gaul
Finished art by Ivy Hansen
Illustrations by Jane Cameron
Typeset by Savage Type Pty Ltd, Brisbane
Printed in Singapore by Toppan Printing Co.

BB 89

The Children's Sports Injuries Handbook

Dr David Kennedy with Peter Fitzgerald

BAY BOOKS

Foreword

This book can be considered essential reading for parents of sporting kids, coaches, teachers and also the medical and paramedical people involved in children's sport.

The authors have combined their respective talents to make a very important contribution to children's sport. With easy, non-clinical style, this book encourages us to read on as our understanding of children's sports medicine unfolds.

Colleagues and friends of David Kennedy respect him as a very dedicated doctor who obviously gains great satisfaction in helping sports people of all types and ages. His experience in sports medicine has been extensive having practised in the USA with professional football and baseball, worked with Australian Rules football teams, the Victorian cricket team and Olympic weightlifters. These experiences, together with his intense interest in younger sports people is testimony to his enthusiasm and commitment to our sporting community.

That Peter Fitzgerald's heart is well and truly behind his work is exemplified by the fact that he once campaigned to popularise the use of helmets for children cyclists.

Among the many important messages emerging throughout the book, two stand out. Firstly, that children are not little adults and must be treated specially as children. Secondly, parents can make a significant contribution to sports injury prevention in their children. This book tells us how to do both. We learn of the relationship of injuries with maturation, the type of sport, the equipment and clothing, playing venues and climatic conditions. We do learn some new medical terms, but they are explained very carefully and a glossary makes it almost impossible to get lost during any description or explanation.

That this book is written to help kids, stands out above all else. It is very clear that the experiences of fatherhood, as well as profession have inspired this fine publication.

Dr Richard Telford
The Australian
Institute of Sport,
Canberra

Contents

FOREWORD

1 FIRST STEPS FOR PARENTS AND COACHES   6

2 GROWTH CENTRE INJURIES   19

3 LITTLE ATHLETICS AND DISTANCE RUNNING   28

4 FOOTBALL: AUSTRALIAN RULES, RUGBY AND SOCCER   43

5 BAT AND BALL SPORTS: CRICKET, BASEBALL, SOFTBALL AND FIELD HOCKEY   59

6 WATER SPORTS: SWIMMING, SURFING, WATER SKIING AND SAILING   67

7 BMX BIKE RIDING, SKATEBOARDING, HORSE RIDING, SNOW-SKIING AND ICE SKATING   75

8 RACQUET SPORTS: TENNIS, SQUASH AND BADMINTON   91

9 NETBALL AND BASKETBALL   103

10 STRENGTH SPORTS: GYMNASTICS AND WEIGHT LIFTING   110

TEN GOLDEN RULES FOR CHILDREN'S SPORT   118

GUIDELINES FOR CHILDREN IN SPORT   120

GLOSSARY   122

QUICK-FIND INJURY INDEX   126

INDEX   126

1 First Steps for Parents and Coaches

Prevention of injury is the cornerstone of this entire book — be the sport through a club, school or even a family activity. Prevention involves thorough preparation for the sport, knowing what to look for and erring on the side of commonsense caution without ruining the fun of things. Children should equate sport with happiness without the fear of getting hurt. You can be positive-minded in quietly organising things for children to unleash all those energies without them resenting an authoritarian heavy hand behind the scenes.

A vast number of children and teenagers are injured each year while playing sport — be it an organised sport or just for fun in the school playground, the local park, the street or an empty parking lot. Children just get carried away with their own immortality when attempting something just a little bit more daring than last time! Most mishaps need never happen. The experience of sports' medical practitioners in Australia, the United States, Canada and Europe is that at least seven out of ten injuries to child athletes could have been avoided with advance knowledge of what part of their anatomy is the most vulnerable.

It must be stressed that sport is relatively safe. The benefits are enormous compared with the risk of injuries which can be greatly minimised. It's my experience that the benefits for children playing sport far outweigh the disadvantages of injury. Childhood is the time when athletic activity can provide the basis for long-term health, physical fitness and nutritional understanding.

Among physical and mental health professionals, there's no question that an appropriately balanced athletic program is a positive factor for general physical and emotional development. We should strongly endorse such sports programs within our schools and communities.

However, as parents and coaches, we should be aware that all athletic events expose the participants to some degree of physical and emotional risk. The answer is to ensure adequate management for maximum safety while permitting active participation.

FIRST STEPS

This book for parents and coaches stresses self-help reliance — with the proviso that you should seek medical attention for serious injuries or when in doubt about the nature of an injury. A knowledge of first aid can be of inestimable value. Parents and coaches should consider doing one of the many excellent courses run by the Red Cross or the St John Ambulance Australia.

> **STOP**
> *When in doubt seek medical attention.*

The St John Ambulance first aid courses have long been recognised as thorough and reliable. In the space of two days you can acquire a senior first aid certificate at little cost. From here, enthusiasts can undergo more advanced courses if they so choose. For further information on the St John Ambulance courses contact:

Adelaide	(08) 274 0444
Brisbane	(07) 52 2092
Hobart	(002) 23 7177
Melbourne	(03) 67 5576
Perth	(09) 277 9999
Darwin	(089) 27 9111
Canberra	(062) 95 8840
Sydney	(02) 212 1088

I have simplified the necessary medical and anatomical terms and the glossary at the back of the book is designed as an easy reference or it can be read in its own right as a summary of sports injury advice.

THE NATURE OF THE PROBLEM

Children cop 40 per cent of all sports injuries. Two-thirds of these involve sprains, strains, contusions, abrasions and lacerations. Only about one in ten are fractures.

This isn't as bad as it may first sound because young children have a tremendous resilience in overcoming injuries such as a sprain which would sideline a teenager or an adult for much longer.

The injury rate jumps as young players and athletes grow older. The competition is keener and the involvement is more physical. Older participants, especially boys, are heavier and stronger.

BOYS, GIRLS AND GROWTH SPURTS

Up to the age of ten, boys and girls are physically similar. The size of their bones and muscles is much the same and they have comparable athletic skills.

FIRST STEPS

Girls start to mature from the age of ten. With adolesence and the start of menstruation, they experience hormonal changes which cause a growth spurt when a girl will grow as much as 10 to 12 centimetres (four or five inches) a year. This gradually ends between the ages of 14 and 16.

Seventy-five per cent of boys will start their growth spurt between the ages of 12 and 15 and the maturational growth period has usually ended by 18. Once the growth spurt slows, muscle mass increases. This usually occurs 6 to 12 months after the growth spurt ends because bones and muscles grow at different rates.

As the muscle tissue develops, the young adolescent boy and girl increase dramatically in strength and weight. Predictably, adolescents who mature earlier are more likely to succeed in most high school sports, particularly the contact sports such as various football codes and basketball.

There is considerable variation between individual maturation times.

There's considerable variation between individual maturation times. Boys generally experience their peak of skeletal growth at about 15 years of age, but some start at 13, while others don't complete this development until 17 or 18. This difference becomes significant when they engage in sporting activities.

CHILDREN ARE NOT LITTLE ADULTS!

One of the most overlooked facts contributing to serious sports injuries is that children are children. They are not little adults. It's therefore essential that doctors, parents and coaches realise this and treat the injuries and the problems that cause such injuries accordingly.

Children whose physical and skeletal patterns mature early will be more powerful and able to compete better than late maturers. This is evident in all studies which have been made of adolescent athletes. Those who mature earlier are stronger and are thus more likely to succeed in state school and high school athletics. Therefore, the problem is how to counsel late maturers about getting the best from their athletic and general sporting prowess. By the time they are 20 years of age, the late maturers will probably be taller and more skilled and stronger than the early maturers. However, while they are young, they shouldn't be mismatched to their physical and emotional detriment.

FIRST STEPS

CHOOSE SPORTS WISELY

A wise selection of sports and recreation activities for our youngsters would go a long way in preventing injuries. The important considerations are to combine the child's ability and physical stature with a realistic and safe sporting achievement goal.

Athletic abilities should be carefully assessed. Unrealistic expectations by coaches, parents and children are a major reason why many children withdraw from physical education and sport.

For equally wrong reasons, handicapped children are frequently excused from sports participation when, in fact, they could benefit more from it than able-bodied children.

Physical mismatching is usually the result of indiscriminately grouping children by age rather than by physical characteristics and body development. These physical mismatches boost the injury rate by as much as 50 per cent — particularly in contact sports.

Opponents of contact sports frequently cite the injury rate as a reason to drop a particular sport from the state or public school curriculum. If, however, the selection methods were improved, injuries could be minimised. The school administrators and sports coaches should look more carefully at the way in which children are selected for participation in such sports. Only then will the injury rate in such contact sports fall dramatically.

Game rules can also be modified for different age groups so as to reduce the risk of injury. Too often, children and parents accept whatever team sports are available at school or in the community. Sometimes, they decide to just opt out. They don't realise there are numerous alternatives available to all children either in individual or team sports.

Conflict can also be caused by the difference between the growth of the body and the technique of the sport itself. For example, a young gymnast with a light, pliant body can be disadvantaged once adolescent growth changes have started. Reappraisals may be necessary as the child grows and develops.

However, it's important to realise that some mechanical factors, in a particular sports event, such as the specialised lifts in weightlifting, apply to all ages. Correct technique is therefore of the greatest importance.

A wise selection of sports helps prevent injuries.

Correct technique is of the greatest importance.

THE PATTERN OF SPORTS IN AUSTRALIA

The pattern of sports in Australia is undergoing sweeping changes and, with that, the pattern of sports injuries. There's a strong trend in Australia for parents and children to go for sports which have an international flavour and representation. That's why we're seeing, to some extent, a decline in the time-honoured sports in this country — cricket and football. Even rugby is limited to Commonwealth countries and France. Netball's world championships are played by several countries, but this also has its limitations. Soccer, on the other hand, is universal. The World Cup stands supreme. Basketball is also an international sport. Australian Rules football and rugby can be very violent sports. I think parents are understandably concerned. For example, head injuries and serious injuries to knees are frequent, which isn't good for the sport. Basketball and soccer tend to be far less violent.

If our community is trying to encourage lifelong physical activity, we need to pay more careful attention to suitable games and recreations offered to school children.

THE MANAGEMENT OF YOUNG SPORTS PARTICIPANTS

General problems in the management of adolescents and young sports participants concern the planning of their training and general life. A long, successful sporting career can be enhanced by maintaining a balanced approach to training and fitness with a good proportion of the different physiological components — speed, stamina, strength and mobility. All should get their fair share of attention. The subtle, mobile young athlete isn't very likely to become a stiff, inactive person in later life.

The all-important warm-up

Warming-up maintains elasticity.

Although children's natural elasticity makes soft-tissue injuries relatively mild and usually quick to heal, it's imperative that young athletes spend time warming-up to maintain this elasticity. A proper warm-up should include:

★ General conditioning exercises that contribute to all aspects of the coming performance, particularly exercises promoting strength, power, speed and/or endurance.
★ Exercises that reproduce the movements of the sport to be played, to achieve a state of neuromuscular and psychological readiness.
★ Exercises to maintain flexibility, such as gradual stretches to reduce the natural resistance and viscosity of the muscles, ligaments and other collagenous tissues.
★ Exercises beginning at a low intensity and gradually building up in intensity.
★ Exercises that are long and intense enough to raise deep body temperature and to break the sweat barrier.

Dealing with stress

Each athlete's ability and motivation should be assessed and realistic expectations defined. Motivation of the child in sport comes from their peers as well as coaches and parents. This is positive feedback. Other children seem to be motivated by fear of failure. This group doesn't handle the stress of participation well.

Assess ability and motivation and define realistic expectations.

Fatigue is also a common problem with the young sports participant. The young adolescent needs adequate sleep and rest. This is a major time for growth which needs its own contribution of energy.

The development of talented young athletes often leads them to gain a distorted view of themselves. Sometimes, this results in a depreciation of their academic performance and personal growth. So, never overlook the importance of achieving a balance between a youngster's academic, athletic and personal achievement.

There are often many pressures at home, in today's environment of domestic money problems and sudden unemployment hitting families. Family breakdowns, separations and divorces also impose tremendous pressures on children.

Stress plays a big part in a wide range of common psychosomatic symptoms such as the stitch and vague abdominal pain or cramp. Sympathetic counselling and co-operation between parents, coaches and school teachers can usually sort out such relatively simple problems about the conflict between schoolwork and examinations on the one hand and sporting pressures on the other.

One of the great tragedies in Western nations is the tendency of adolescent sports participants to quit their sport when they leave school. This must largely be a reflection of unsatisfactory sporting achievements or the environment in which they participate.

STEPS IN MINIMISING INJURY

The injury rate can be substantially reduced by proper preventive measures. Prerequisites to injury prevention are appropriate and adequate conditioning and the careful fitting of athletic gear and equipment according to individual needs.

Good conditioning, gear and equipment are essential.

On a national scale prevention of sporting injuries would be boosted by selecting youngsters for sports on a more scientific basis, according to their anatomical and physiological suitability for the widely different sports available. Unfortunately, some parents and coaches have such a rush of blood

FIRST STEPS

to the head that they seem incapable of being objective about physical criteria such as body size and development.

The real answer to sporting injuries in young children and adolescents lies in an analysis of the individual's sporting style. The prowess of individual participants will largely depend on the correction of their faults.

This doesn't require expert knowledge of all sports by school administrators, parents, coaches and doctors. Rather, it calls for an alertness to the possibility of sporting inefficiency and recognising that the correct approach to the problem suggests its own answer.

Various European studies on young athletic participants identified at least 70 per cent of injuries as being preventable (for example, joint instability, muscle tightness or lack of flexibility, inadequate rehabilitation after injury and neglect of equipment or the rules). Correction of these factors in the studies cut the injury rate by 75 per cent compared with the control group, that is, the uncorrected teams.

At least 70 per cent of injuries are preventable.

★ Carefully selecting and fitting all sporting gear and equipment also minimises the probability of injury. Your aim should always be to buy the best possible equipment within your budget — and then correctly wear or use it.

★ The continued improvement of all types of playing surfaces, facilities and athletic equipment is an important factor in reducing injury rates, particularly in young children and adolescents. Also, careful treatment and consideration of the injured athlete will help considerably in preventing further injury and ensuring that permanent problems don't develop.

★ Unfamiliarity with many fundamentals of the game can cause both a host of sporting problems and stress in children and young adolescents. This can result in them being awkward and accident-prone in situations which have injury-provoking potential. Participants should, therefore, spend time becoming familiar with the rules and fundamentals of the sporting activity.

★ Pre-conditioning of the young athlete is important in developing strength, endurance, flexibility and speed so that the participant is able to meet and surmount hazardous situations. A tackle, or a push from the side, may move a particular joint beyond its limit resulting in an injury to the capsule, ligament or adjacent muscle and tendon. Therefore, calisthenics and mobility exercises are of the greatest importance in the preparation for sporting activities. The increase in flexibility and range of joint movement coupled with the strength of supporting muscles enables the young participant to withstand more severe strain, impact and twisting than previously.

FIRST STEPS

UNDERSTANDING EQUIPMENT
Strapping for prevention and strapping an injury

It's a common fallacy that strapping can protect against injury, regardless of the circumstances. It should always be remembered that protective devices have their limitations and that, occasionally, they may even encourage the injury risk of some sports.

When dealing with a young player who has an injury to a particular joint, and you're deciding whether to apply a bandage to that joint to give mechanical support or protection to enable a return to the sporting activity, the decision must be made on the basis of sound anatomical principles.

The most fundamental question whenever strapping is concerned is to consider the diagnosis of the problem and the permitted function of that joint following the injury.

For example, if you have just pulled a muscle which has now become swollen because of bleeding in that muscle and it isn't fit to support normal movements, you should never try to perform that movement with the assistance of strapping or bandages applied to the injured muscle. No amount of strapping will be safe. It's bad medicine and psychologically unsound to allow a convalescing young player to resume attempts to play until he, or she, is anatomically sound. That is, the injury has healed with a resumption of full function to the area. Usually, when this has occurred, the participant doesn't require any additional mechanical support or the application of bandages or of non-stretch tape.

Protective devices have their limitations.

Helmets

Another major misconception is that a sports helmet will give the participant absolute protection from head and neck injuries. The helmet may just not be strong enough to survive some severe impact. On the other hand, the helmet may be designed to remain unbroken — but not able to absorb the shock sufficiently to prevent injury to the wearer.

FIRST STEPS

Non-stretch tape

There's considerable value in using non-stretch tape which may be applied to joints. It does two things.

1. MECHANICAL SUPPORT

A small amount of mechanical support may be given to ligament structures.

A classic example of such protection is the U-shaped stirrup applied to an ankle joint following a sprain. The simple stirrup allows the hinge movement of the ankle to occur with minimal restriction. This adds support to the ligaments on either side of the ankle during twisting and turning movements.

2. ENHANCED STABILITY

The awareness of the joint to its surrounding circumstances (known as 'proprioception') may be enhanced by using non-stretch tape applied to a joint.

For example, when the foot is planted on the ground and moves slightly, this nervous awareness of the joint sends messages to the brain which, in turn, sends a message to the muscles which support that particular joint. This results in the enhancing of the joint's functional stability when load-bearing forces are applied.

CATEGORISING SPORTS INJURIES

Sports injuries can be categorised into two kinds: trauma injuries and overuse injuries.

Trauma injuries are those involving contact with other players, equipment or other obstacles during the participation in a particular sporting activity.

Overuse injuries, which account for about one-third of all reported injuries, are simply due to the locomotor system — that is bones, joints and muscles — showing dynamic symptoms of stress. In other words, an athlete may excessively stress either a muscle or a capsule lining of a joint in a sporting activity by constantly and repetitively using it over a prolonged period of time. It is also possible if a muscle or joint is being used repetitively and intensively over a short period. This constant, repetitive use causes those tissues to break down and malfunction which means limitations to certain movements.

Overuse injuries can vary from muscle stiffness to the stretching of a tendon or ligament due to unaccustomed exercise or prolonged repetitive exercise. They can also include a whole variety of injuries from those involving the soft tissues to those involving the bone itself, including the classic stress fracture.

A stress fracture is caused by repetitive stress to a bone, resulting in the breakdown of the bone's normal structure. This is in contrast to a fracture that occurs because of trauma — usually an intense force applied to the bone which results in the immediate breakdown of the architectural structure.

The essential point about overuse injuries is that no one but the participant is responsible for the overuse injury and that this breakdown — whether it involves muscles, tendons, ligaments or bones — relates only to the mechanical movements undertaken.

The age pattern of sport is gradually changing so that many young children and adolescents are today being subjected to loads far greater than what was once thought acceptable, in terms of mechanics of movement involving particular bone and muscle structures.

Ambitious parents and coaches don't easily see why their children should be 'second rate'. They simply don't understand the many mechanical factors operating in different sports. These parents and coaches often don't understand that the risks their children take in certain sports could be sensibly minimised without lessening the enjoyment and the chance of winning.

An understanding of the varying mechanical stresses which are applied to the locomotor system in different sports, and an understanding of how preventive measures can help avoid such injuries, are two of the keys to successful management of the sports-injured child.

THE VITAL IMPORTANCE OF RICE

The cornerstone of all sports injuries is RICE. This is the most important immediate treatment for all athletic injuries whether the child has pulled a muscle from a strained ligament or broken a bone. The letters in the acronym stand for:

★ *Rest*. This is essential because continued exercise, or extended physical activity, could extend the length of time the injury persists. Use of the injured part should stop the minute it's hurt and a sling or crutches used if necessary.

★ *Ice*. This decreases the bleeding from the injured blood vessels by causing them to contract. The more blood that collects in a wound, the longer it takes to heal.

★ *Compression*. This limits swelling which, if uncontrolled, could retard healing. Following damage to a tissue, blood and fluid from the surrounding tissues bleed into the damaged area and distend the tissue. That's all swelling is. Swelling can be useful in some instances, particularly if the skin is broken and the area has become infected. Antibodies then collect in the swelling to kill the germs. But, if the skin hasn't been broken, antibodies may not be necessary and the swelling can delay healing.

★ *Elevation*. Elevation of the injured area to above the level of the heart assists the return of blood to the heart by using gravity to help drain excess fluid from the damaged area.

FIRST STEPS

RICE: STEP-BY-STEP PROCEDURES

Because swelling usually starts within seconds of an injury, start RICE immediately. Don't wait for a doctor's advice.

First place a wet towel over the injured area. Then apply ice in the form of an ice pack, ice chips or ice cubes in a wet towel. Never apply the ice directly to the skin, or in a plastic ice pack, because it can cause the skin to burn and become painful.

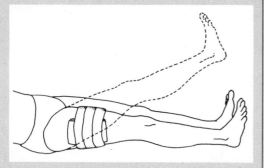

RICE, the cornerstone of early treatment for muscle and joint injuries.

For compression, wrap an elastic bandage firmly over the ice around the injured part. Be careful not to wrap the area so tightly that you cut off the blood supply. The signs of a shut-off blood supply are numbness, cramping and further pain. If any of these occur, immediately unwrap the injured area. Otherwise, leave the ice pack and the bandage in place for approximately 30 minutes.

Elevate the injured area so that it is above the level of the heart.

Next, to allow the skin to become warm and the blood to recirculate, unwrap the area for 15 minutes. Repeat this procedure for three hours. If the area continues to swell, or pain increases, immediately check with a doctor if you haven't already done so.

With a severe injury, you can follow the RICE program for 48 to 72 hours. Further treatment depends on the type of tissue which has been injured.

WHEN TO SEE A DOCTOR

If you are concerned about the injury and are unsure about whether the child should see a doctor, I would recommend you follow these guidelines:

★ Pain. Any injury which causes severe pain should be seen by a doctor because pain is nature saying that something is seriously amiss. When it's severe, you should 'listen'. Also, if the pain in a bone or joint persists for more than two weeks, then these tissues are the ones in which the most serious injuries have occurred.

★ All joint injuries should be seen by a doctor. This also goes for any injuries which haven't healed within two weeks. They should be checked for structural abnormalities. Injuries to a joint involve damage to a capsule and possibly ligaments. If not treated promptly, these injuries have the potential to become permanent and cause significant future problems. Any joint injury should be immobilised until seen by a doctor.

★ If function has been lost. If the child cannot move a limb or a joint (such as an ankle or a finger) the injury should be assessed as soon as possible.

★ Any injury which appears to be infected, which is manifested by pus, discolouration of the skin, swollen lymph nodes

See a doctor with any injury which causes severe pain, hasn't healed within three weeks or which is infected.

FIRST STEPS

or fever, can lead to serious complications if uncontrolled. Generally, antibiotics bring quick relief.

These are only simple guidelines to whether a sports injury should be seen by a doctor. Every injury is an individual event and every situation is unique. If you're unsure about whether a doctor should be seen, commonsense is the best guide.

HOW LONG WILL IT TAKE TO RECOVER?

The golden rule in orthopaedics is three days, three weeks or three months. That was almost holy writ in my medical training. But I've learned through hard experience that life and medicine are not that simple. The doctor and the patient should always expect the unexpected!

Healing time mainly depends on blood supply because the blood brings the elements necessary for the healing to occur.

★ Nutrients. Think of the injury as a remodelling job. Nutrients are the building materials for healing.
★ Oxygen. This is the energy source for the healing project. I tell my patients that you can't have fire without oxygen. Similarly, the body can't heal without oxygen.
★ Inflammatory cells. These are the workers in the healing process. They carry away the old blood and the dead tissue. They also fight off infection by assembling the building blocks. Unfortunately, the best they can do is a slick patch-up job. Most body tissue, except the liver, heals with scar tissue. The larger the injury, the bigger the scar. It's this biological fact that explains why the body never really totally forgets an injury.

WHEN SHOULD ASPIRIN BE USED?

Aspirin's benefits are often not realised.

★ It is an excellent pain-killer or analgesic.
★ It is an effective anti-inflammatory medication.
★ It quickly reduces fever.
★ It is a safe medication.

I use aspirin mainly for its pain-relieving and anti-inflammatory effectiveness. I immediately use with patients suffering irritated tendons (tendinitis), irritated nerves (neuritis) or swollen joints.

If you're giving a child too much aspirin, their stomach will 'speak up' with heartburn. The best prevention is to take an aspirin with meals.

After absorption, aspirin is rapidly distributed through all body tissues. It is excreted from the body mainly by the kidneys. About 50 per cent of a given dose is eliminated within 24 hours.

Rehabilitation should start as soon as the swelling stops. That means that within 48 hours after an injury, you should be working with a physiotherapist or trainer.

WHEN CAN SPORT BE RESUMED?

Here are my guidelines:

★ If the injured area hurts at rest, it shouldn't be exercised.
★ As soon as the injured part doesn't hurt at rest, it may be exercised minimally. That means *slowly*. If the pain resumes stop exercising. Listen to those body signals!
★ As soon as the exercise can be handled without pain, increase the intensity and the duration of the exercise program. Expect a little aching. But remember to stop immediately sharp pain starts.

When recovering from any athletic injury, it's important to maintain cardiovascular fitness. Thus, if a child has an injured ankle, encourage them to perform a sport that doesn't require strenuous use of the ankle. For example, try swimming. If it is a wrist injury, try bicycling. It only takes about six weeks to lose cardiovascular endurance. Any exercise will be of more benefit than resting in bed or sitting in a warm bath.

If a child doesn't quickly rehabilitate after an injury, their muscles will remain in a weakened condition. Even if they return to full sports activity, the muscles will remain weak and the child will subconsciously favour the injured limb.

The body will simply not feel right until full strength has returned. Also, a child will be very vulnerable to reinjury. In a weakened condition, an injured part simply cannot protect itself against the stress of sports participation.

Growth Centre Injuries

2

There are many specific injuries to children and to young adolescents involving the growth aspects of the locomotor system. Any injury to a growth centre can be serious. It's growth centres which are the mechanism for growth of the long and flat bones of the body. Injuries to the growth centres can stunt growth or result in permanent joint deformity.

An injury can happen in many ways — a fall, a twist, a turn. The growth centre can be fractured — that is, broken, compressed or torn. Some, or all of the growth cells may die and this can lead to altered patterns of growth development.

The injury may heal without any long-term deformity. Growth may be slowed temporarily until the fracture, or compression, of the growth centre has healed. Normal growth then continues. However, the growth centre can stop growing altogether if it has been significantly damaged.

Any injury to a growth centre can be serious.

The potential for deformity resulting from an injury to the growth centre is tremendous. Take for example, an injury to the growth centre of the thigh bone — the femur. While the injured centre is healing, the other leg is growing and this can mean a difference of one to two centimetres a year. In the case of a 12-year-old boy, this could account for one leg being three or four centimetres shorter at the end of the growth period.

Sometimes, growth centres are only partially injured. This is an even more difficult medical situation because the growth centres usually only cause part of the bone to grow. In this case, if the child's bone grows out of line, then it will be angular or crooked.

In the lower leg, above the ankle or in the lower arm above the wrist, there will be two bones growing. If only one is injured, then the effect of the growth discrepancy and the normal growth of the non-injured bone must be looked at for their effect on the joint's function.

In a rapidly growing young adolescent, the injury to a knee from a side tackle is much more likely to be a growth centre fracture than a ligament injury.

A ligament injury would be more common in a fully grown person. But, in a young adolescent, the essential thing to remember is that a ligament is stronger than a growth centre.

GROWTH CENTRE INJURIES

These growth centre injuries are usually seen under two circumstances. Sometimes, the child is brought to a doctor with a routine fracture or a joint problem and the bones are X-rayed. When the bones are compared with the healthy bone, or joint, there's an irregularity on the X-ray showing up in the growth centre. The other common way a child presents for treatment is when the parent notices a small limp or when a small bone is growing crookedly.

Injuries to growth centres, and joints, present very different problems for the young adolescent. An injury may result to the joint surface cartilage and the maturing bone beneath the surface. This is called an 'intra-articular fracture' and is usually identified by careful X-ray examination of the joint. Invariably, such a fracture will require an operative procedure for proper re-estabishment of a smooth joint surface.

At the time of early adolescence, children can commonly present with a unique growth plate injury known as a 'slipped epiphysis'. This is an injury to a growth centre. The most frequent is a slipped capital femoral epiphysis, that is, the ball of the hip joint becomes displaced.

This may happen gradually, or suddenly, during a sporting or physical event. The young adolescent is usually of a chubby body type and surgery may be required to prevent further slipping of the epiphysis. There's a 25 per cent chance of this happening to the other hip. Therefore, careful observation is important.

An 'avulsion fracture' is the name doctors give to fractures of the growth centres of flat bones. The most frequent sites of avulsions are the growth centres of the pelvic bone.

The large muscles of the back and abdomen extend into the top of the pelvis bone at the growth centre. Children and young adolescents who participate in sports that demand sudden twisting manoeuvres frequently sustain avulsion injuries.

GROWTH CENTRE INJURIES

OVERUSE SYNDROMES

Overuse syndromes in children, and young adolescents, are common. They happen when a child, or a young adolescent, exercises or trains too much. Frequently, the tissue cannot tolerate the strain and becomes injured. It's not unusual to see young swimmers who train six hours a day, weightlifters who train twice a day six days a week and gymnasts who even live away from home with their coaches so they have more time to train! However, there's an upper limit to the amount of work that even a highly conditioned body can perform.

Never be carried away with enthusiasm. It's always wise to keep a commonsense perspective of a child's physical limits, rather than expecting them to be able to achieve miracle performances.

Some individuals have a genetic predisposition to an overuse syndrome. In others, it may be hastened by lax ligaments or capsules supporting a joint.

There are several levels, or grades, of overuse syndromes. In the mild grade, a child normally complains of a slight ache during exercise or sporting activities. Sometimes, the pain continues for a short time after the exercise ends. X-rays don't usually show any tissue changes.

In the next grade of overuse syndrome, the pain occurs during the performance, shortens participation time and continues after the performance has been stopped. X-rays show early changes of bone and growth centres, particularly when compared with normal tissues.

In the third grade of overuse syndrome, the pain is significant during the performance as well as afterwards. It can last for many hours after the physical activity has ceased. The injury site swells and there's a difference in motion between the injured and the uninjured limb. X-ray changes are identifiable. This is usually in the form of excessive bone development or bone fragment development. At this particular level of overuse syndrome, it's important to understand that sporting activities have to be suspended for six to eight weeks and sometimes even longer. Sometimes, it's wise to apply a splint or cast to the limb or joint to promote rest.

In the most severe form of overuse syndrome, the child is unable to perform for an extended period because of persistent pain in the injured area. After exercise, or stopping sporting activities, the pain lasts for more than 24 hours. X-rays show definite changes and usually the child, or young adolescent, has lost a full range of motion. In this final stage, the youngster has significant problems and it's best to advise rest for several months and, frequently, to change sports.

Keep a commonsense perspective of a child's physical limits.

LEVEL ONE

LEVEL TWO

LEVEL THREE

LEVEL FOUR

GROWTH CENTRE INJURIES

It's important to listen to children and to encourage them to speak up when they're hurt. All too often, parents, coaches and team-mates encourage the injured youngster to play despite pain. This short-sighted attitude is almost guaranteed to lead to the development of level three and four overuse syndromes.

Pain is nature's way of telling your child that something is wrong.

Pain is nature's way of telling your child that something is wrong. When it speaks, you should heed its advice! One of the classic examples of an overuse stress syndrome in children and young adolescents is the development of acute tendonitis in long-distance running.

The Australian Sports' Medicine Federation, in conjunction with guidelines from the American College of Sports Medicine, has laid down special guidelines to reduce overuse syndromes. (See page 120 .) The guidelines particularly apply to long-distance running involving children and young adolescents. A child encouraged to participate at a higher rate than the recommended guidelines is at extreme risk of developing an overuse syndrome.

The current treatment of overuse syndrome in children, and young adolescents, is prevention or early recognition. The tragedy is when a level three or four problem is diagnosed and the sad news has to be broken to the child and the parents. What a waste when it was all avoidable if caught early enough.

AVULSIONS

Avulsions are true fractures.

Avulsions involve much more than a muscle pull or strain. They are true fractures. The significance of diagnosing them correctly is that the healing time is significantly longer than with a muscle pull or strain.

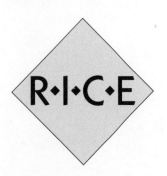

An avulsion can take two to six months to heal. In general, it's not necessary to operate on an avulsion injury. The best treatment is RICE, rest and protection, carefully increasing rehabilitation and a cautious return to sporting activity.

GROWTH CENTRE INJURIES

OSTEOCHONDROSES

Osteochondroses are a group of disorders which occur in the growing areas of bone. They are simply a non-infectious interruption of the blood supply resulting in injured tissue in that area.

It usually begins with some single, or repetitive, injury (known as an 'episode trauma') to a bone or joint. Frequently, this occurs with overuse syndromes. Such situations affect the blood supply to the developing bone.

The symptoms usually follow excessive physical demands of sports participation and are most frequently identified during these early stages of growth development.

Any unusual compressive, or shearing, force may produce some change in the shape of the bone-cartilage unit or interfere with the area's blood supply. This changes its development and also its X-ray image.

Early diagnosis of an osteochondrosis usually means healing without major deformity or disability. If it isn't easily identified, then it's possible that the symptoms will continue long-term with joint deformity and eventually impairment and disability.

Usually, doctors grade the severity of osteochondroses from grades one to four. Generally, the younger the child and the higher the grade, the more concern doctors have about the ultimate outcome.

There are two kinds of osteochondroses of childhood. Legg-Perthes syndrome is osteochondrosis of the femoral head that is, the ball of the hip joint. Secondly, there's Kohler's syndrome — osteochondrosis of the navicular bone of the foot.

Osteochondroses are non-infectious interruptions of the blood supply.

Legg-Perthes syndrome

Legg-Perthes syndrome usually occurs in children between four and eight years of age. The specific cause is unknown, but it's related to the restriction of blood supply to the head of the femur — the thigh bone — which becomes significantly altered with continued repetitive running and jumping. The child's complaint is usually one of the following:

★ Pain about the hip and thigh.
★ A painless limp.
★ A mild limp with pain localising on the inner side of the knee.

GROWTH CENTRE INJURIES

The complaint of knee pain when the problem is in the hip is common.

The complaint of knee pain, when the problem is in the hip, occurs all too often in children. A very important rule of thumb for medical students is, when a child is complaining of knee pain, to automatically question and X-ray the hip because of referred pain to the region of the knee joint.

Non-surgical and surgical treatment are both considerations for the treatment of Legg-Perthes syndrome. In early diagnosis, common non-surgical treatment with a brace will frequently produce satisfactory results. An operation may be necessary for a child with a long-standing history of, or advanced, deformity with progressive X-ray changes. Any child with a diagnosis of Legg-Perthes syndrome will probably be kept from participating in running and jumping sports for between 12 to 24 months.

Kohler's syndrome

Kohler's syndrome is a similar process which occurs in the tarsal-navicular bone of the foot. The tarsal-navicular is in the inner part of the middle of the foot.

The initial treatment is rest. The limitation of activities or immobilisation of the foot in a splint or cast for six to eight weeks is usually sufficient to resolve the problem.

Osgood-Schlatter's syndrome

The most common form of osteochondrosis in early adolescence is Osgood-Schlatter's syndrome. It affects the front part of the upper tibia, just below the knee joint. This area can be felt as a bump, four to six centimetres below the kneecap.

When this cartilage converts to bone, or there's some repetitive stress on the attachment of the patella from the thigh muscles, a series of micro-fractures are created. This interrupts the normal blood supply and the normal conversion of the cartilage to bone resulting in a tender bump. The major symptoms are localised pain and pain when pressure is applied to the bump.

The young athlete will typically complain of pain after activities such as running, jumping and kneeling. This is a condition which will heal when growth is completed. Until then, it's important to advise the young athlete to stay away from certain sporting activities that increase the pain. In some cases, it's necessary to apply a cast for six to eight weeks to aid the healing and to prevent further irritation and disruption of the blood supply.

Scheuermann's disease

Other osteochondroses occur in the vertebral bodies of the spine during adolescence and account for postural deformities such as Scheuermann's disease, a similar complaint.

Once again, the key to success is early diagnosis, an appropriate change of activity and prescribed exercises or the use of a cast or external bracing support.

The bone surfaces which form joints are covered with a glistening, white cartilage which is very slippery. Joint surface cartilage can be easily damaged. It can happen with a fall, turn, twist or tackle. The cartilage, nourished and lubricated by joint fluid, has considerable elasticity and recovers from denting remarkably well.

Joint surface cartilage can be easily damaged.

Osteochondritis dissecans

Osteochondritis dissecans is a defect in the joint-bone cartilage of any synovial joint — the knee, wrist, ankle or elbow. An X-ray of the area looks like a small excavation out of the joint surface. In time, the piece may loosen and cause pain. The dissecans refers to a dissection of a loose piece from the surface of the joint.

In children, the dissecans usually remains seated in the divot — the excavated area. However, in athletes aged between 12 and 16, the divot sometimes falls free. When the piece does fall free into the joint, it is called a 'joint mouse' because it may wander around the joint.

In osteochondritis dissecans, the pain usually starts when the cartilage piece loosens from its bed. The movement of the piece causes the pain. If the child doesn't move the joint, no pain is created. Sometimes, a plain or regular X-ray of the joint doesn't identify the surface of the joint accurately enough.

In such cases, dye may have to be put into the joint to outline the joint surface and, in cases of osteochondritis dissecans, can outline the fragment and the bone surface. This test is called an 'arthrogram'.

The status of a fragment can also be determined with an arthroscope, a joint telescope that can peer inside a narrow opening in the joint. This type of procedure is usually performed under general anaesthetic.

GROWTH CENTRE INJURIES

In young children, the treatment of osteochondritis dissecans is rest. Sometimes, this means a splint or a cast. Rest usually works in 99 per cent of cases because the cartilage is still growing and usually covers the divot. There's usually no lasting deformity. Osteochondritis dissecans is usually a problem of diagnosis, not treatment.

In the 12- to 16-year-old age group, sometimes a splint or cast is recommended, but this would be better avoided if possible. If the fragment is present on a plain X-ray and the surface is intact, then the best way to proceed is to restrict sporting activities. Usually, this means three to six months of no sports. Sometimes, a splint may be applied to the joint to restrict motion. But, again this is better avoided because the muscles around the joint will reduce in size and strength and this in turn slows rehabilitation and a return to physical activities.

I don't use cortisone injections, radiation or dietary changes. I have found they don't significantly help. Surgery must be considered if, after six months, the patient still experiences pain and the X-rays are unchanged. In young people, whose joints are still growing, it makes sense to try to stimulate the healing of the fragment. The operation stimulates the blood supply from the bone to the fragment.

If the athlete is skeletally mature, and has completed bone growth, my experience is that it's almost biologically impossible for the cartilage to heal itself. Accordingly, an operation is the most effective solution.

Developmental lesions

Without apparent reason, some children develop irregularities of bone during their growing process that result in minor developmental abnormalities. This growth irregularity occurs in approximately 20 per cent of the population.

Fibrocystic lesions

Osteochondromas

The two most common are firstly, benign fibrocystic lesions which grow near the growth centres. In the majority of children, these occur just above the knee joint. Secondly, there are osteochondromas which are small projections of bone that extend away from the shaft of the bone. Sometimes they touch nerves or interfere with muscle function and cause pain.

In most instances, these developmental lesions are identified on an X-ray taken because of some other problem. In most cases, they disappear or don't cause structural or physical interference. The best treatment is, therefore, instruction about the lesion. The child is usually permitted to continue with sporting activities.

GROWTH CENTRE INJURIES

In a rare instance, an osteochondroma will cause local discomfort or may interfere with a nerve or muscle function. In those cases, it may be necessary to surgically remove the abnormal bone growth.

Other developmental lesions that may be of greater significance are tumours of the extremities. Not all tumours are malignant. However, even benign tumours can increase in size and may cause weakness and pain in the extremity.

Tumours and tumorous conditions of bone are most frequently brought to the attention of parents and physicians by a recent injury. In many cases, it's implied that the injury is the cause of the tumour or tumorous condition. In reality, the bone has been weakened by the underlying process to the point where a small stress or trauma results in a mild fracture. This in turn causes the pain. When investigating the cause of the pain, X-rays reveal the abnormality of the bone consistent with some tumour or tumorous condition. In some cases, the tumour may be a benign lesion such as a bone cyst. The cyst has increased in size to a point where just throwing, or kicking, a ball creates enough stress to result in a fracture. Such fractures are known as 'pathological fractures'.

Don't diagnose problems only in terms of sporting injuries.

Other times, the lesion may be caused by a bone tumour, growing within the bone or one that has spread to an area of bone from another site. Again, the bone is generally weakened to the extent that mild trauma results in a pathological fracture. This causes the pain and brings the child to the attention of the physician.

Thus, whenever a child complains of pain, or appears to have sustained even an insignificant injury, you should listen! If questions remain, see the school trainer, nurse or doctor. Always remember that children, and young adolescents, who participate in sports are not immune from disease and tumours and other problems that afflict the general population. Parents, coaches and doctors shouldn't fall into the trap of diagnosing the problems which affect a young athlete only in terms of injuries which can happen on the sporting field.

STOP
When a child complains of pain, listen!

3

Little Athletics and Distance Running

The emphasis should be on the pleasure of involvement.

Children are not little adults! That statement is never truer than when discussing running in Little Athletics. The emphasis on running, particularly long-distance running, by children should never be on the duration or intensity of the activities. Rather, it should be in the pleasure of involvement in a variety of activities as well as the development and appreciation of skills in throwing, running and jumping, all of which can be gained with the wide variety of excellent activities provided by Little Athletics.

The main sports injuries problems occur when there's overuse of various parts of the body due to excessive demands placed upon it. These excessive demands commonly include the intensity of the action performed, together with the duration of the stresses. This is particularly so in long-distance running.

Any problems with overuse injuries can be kept to a minimum, provided these demands are monitored and controlled, particularly during the child's growth and development period.

OVER-REALISTIC EXPECTATIONS BY PARENTS

When there's a strong competitive element in such sports, problems can arise more often with parents and coaches than with the children.

Without realising it, parents are often trying to fulfil their own desires and ambitions through their child's participation in competitive sports.

It's the taking part in the sporting activity and the development of basic skills — rather than winning or losing — which are the most important things in the early formative period of a child's development in physical activities.

LITTLE ATHLETICS

Interestingly, when children are asked about their reasons for participating in physical activities, the competitive element is often not included in their top three or four priorities. Most important for the children is the feeling of participation with their team-mates in physical activities which help them integrate within a particular social group. It is only when asked about the element of competition that many children reply that success in sport is important to them to fulfil the expectations of their parents and their coaches.

As adults, we should be more aware of our children's desires and expectations and respond to them when developing and organising their physical activities. The goals should be participation by our children in many and varied physical activities. Little Athletics can be an excellent vehicle for this, provided the emphasis is on the child's growth and development with an ever increasing acquisition of desired skills rather than the ambitious pursuit of medals on the victory dais at all costs. Success will come naturally when the child has physically and emotionally matured.

The goal should be participation in many and varied activities.

THE IMPORTANCE OF EVENTS BEING WELL ORGANISED

If you have ever been to a Little Athletics competition, you can understand what an organisational nightmare it can be with so many small children in such an enclosed area performing such a variety of physical activities simultaneously! It's therefore imperative that the organisation is of a high standard because accidents can easily happen in such situations.

It's important to make sure that the various events are not staged in such a way as to increase the risk of injury from flying objects or from falling over hurdles or other pieces of equipment.

Carefully check the venue for hazards

Tight co-ordination is necessary by the organising committee to schedule the particular sporting activities to reduce the risk of serious injuries.

LITTLE ATHLETICS

The arena should be checked for damage and protruding objects.

The sand must be dry.

The actual arena, including the track, should always be checked for areas of damage which could cause runners to twist their ankles or fall over and sustain cuts or bruises. The arena's inner surface should also be checked for protruding objects such as sprinkler systems or other pieces of equipment thoughtlessly left lying about. These can cause serious injury to participants concentrating more on their activities than on what may be under their feet. With such events as the long jump and the triple jump, the run-up should also be checked for damage. Most importantly, the landing pit should also be thoroughly inspected to make sure the sand is raked and that there are no hidden objects concealed in the landing area. It's also very important that the sand is dry. If it's been extremely wet before the competition, and almost muddy in the landing area, then the staging of that particular event should be cancelled. Serious injuries can occur to the knees and to the hips of competitors landing in a very wet, sloppy pit area.

I had an example of such an incident when working in Toronto, Canada. I was at the Sports Clinic with Dr Robert Jackson when a young boy arrived with a badly swollen knee. He related how he had been long jumping the previous day when he had landed and slipped in the wet pit and felt his knee hyperextend — that is, to go beyond full straightening. He was certain something major had snapped. An extensive examination showed he had damaged his posterior cruciate ligament — one of the ligaments in the middle of the knee at the back. He had, in fact, sustained a complete rupture of the posterior cruciate ligament as well as damage to the menisci — the cartilages — on both sides of the knee. After performing an arthroscopy, his knee was placed in a plaster cast to heal over six to eight weeks.

As we left the operating room, Dr Jackson was still perplexed about how such a serious injury could occur. The answer wasn't long in coming.

We were reading a newspaper while waiting in the surgeons' room for the next patient to come from the ward. There, on the back page, was a photograph of this boy long jumping in the pouring rain and landing in this pit that was awash with water and sloppy sand. The photograph was a classic illustration of his leg hyperextending as his foot hit and slipped forward approximately two feet without any grip in the sand. It was immediately clear how this serious injury had happened.

STOP
Postpone events if it is too hot or too wet.

I must therefore re-emphasise the importance of an awareness of climatic conditions when staging events, particularly Little Athletics. Serious injuries can be avoided by deferring certain events depending on the climatic conditions — whether it be water on the track or in the landing pit.

LITTLE ATHLETICS

The other climatic condition to be wary of is extremely hot or humid weather especially when attempting to stage middle- to long-distance running events.

Landing pit hazards are also overlooked with dire results every year for high jumpers. Such pits are usually constructed with large rubber pontoons placed together to provide a softly cushioned landing when performing the high jump, or with older athletes, the pole vault. It's very important to have a marshal, or organiser, maintaining the effectiveness of the rubber pontoons or mattresses.

Maintain the effectiveness of rubber pontoons or mattresses.

There are numerous examples of serious injuries being caused by inadequate divisioning of the rubber pontoons resulting in an unnecessarily heavy landing. The most important thing is to make sure that the rubber pontoons don't separate in the middle — particularly in the area where the athletes usually land.

I have experienced several cases where a young athlete has successfully cleared the bar — only to disappear between the pontoons, with only his feet visible!

As luck would have it, there were no serious injuries but it's inevitable that, unless such risks are minimised with more care and thoughtfulness, serious injuries will occur to the back or legs. Talented young athletes are too valuable to subject to such unnecessary risks.

LONG-DISTANCE RUNNING

Extensive experience in staging long-distance running events for children has led to many important guidelines being established by the Australian Sports' Medicine Federation and the American College of Sports' Medicine. All of these have the underlying truth that children are not little adults. Certain stresses which adults may be able to handle in relation to long-distance running may be beyond children. I believe that children under the age of 12 shouldn't run in long-distance events beyond 5 to 10 kilometres.

Children are not little adults!

In my opinion, the staging of marathons for young children is fraught with danger. This becomes even more critical in the staging of long-distance running events in warmer, humid weather.

For events involving children running for five kilometres or more, organisers must be aware of the temperature and humidity. If the temperature is beyond 27 degrees Celsius, serious consideration should be given to postponing the event.

Children under the age of 12 shouldn't run in long-distance events beyond 5 to 10 kilometres.

LITTLE ATHLETICS

Provide water and drinks every half to one kilometre along the route of an event five kilometres or more.

It's important to understand that children have a significantly different ratio of body surface area to body mass when compared with adults. This means that children have a larger surface area through which to lose water and salt in the form of perspiration at a greater rate than adults. Simply put, kids cook quicker! This is the body's way of attempting to cool its core temperature which rises in hot weather, particularly when performing a strenuous physical act such as running. Thus, a young child can dehydrate at a greater rate than an adult in the same climatic conditions when performing proportionately the same physical activities.

It's therefore vital that rehydration stations, providing water and drinks for participants, be placed at every half to one kilometre along the route of an event of five kilometres or more. An equally important requirement is that first aid stations, manned by qualified personnel with training in the management of dehydration and other running problems, be placed at every two kilometres.

STOP
The emphasis should be on fun, growth and development.

By following these clear and simple guidelines when staging a running event for young children, potentially fatal situations can be easily avoided. The emphasis in the participation of young children in physical activity should be on fun, growth and development. It is certainly not an opportunity for parents to match their children in stressful situations in an atmosphere of intense competitiveness.

THE IMPORTANCE OF THE RIGHT SHOES

Injury prevention measures in distance running should logically start with running shoes. A good pair doesn't necessarily mean an expensive pair.

The important guidelines when selecting a new pair of running shoes, or when considering whether an old pair should be replaced, are firstly that the shoes should be well fitting — not too tight and not too loose. Secondly, they should also have an element of flexibility in the mid-sole. This can be tested by bending the shoe back towards the heel with your hand. You should be able to do this without excessive force to about 50 degrees from the horizontal. The mid-sole of the shoe should be firm while at the same time allowing enough flexibility for variation of movement during the running phases. The shape of the child's feet should also be observed because most feet curve slightly inwards towards the toe.

Just to make life interesting, sometimes a foot may be absolutely straight. There are shoes which are made straight and lasted so that the sole is in a straight line. Alternatively, there are shoes which bend slightly towards the inside, particularly in that part of the shoe towards the toe box.

If you remove the insole from the shoe, you will see that some shoes are made in a style which is called 'split-lasted' in which the shoe's last is split and then sewn together. Other shoes, are 'board-lasted'. Because this results in a stiffer shoe, they should be used by heavier runners while split-lasted shoes are better suited to lighter runners.

There should also be adequate room in the toe box for all the toes to fit without cramping. Otherwise, blisters can form, particularly on the inner side of the big toe and also on the outer side of the little toe.

Probably, the most important consideration in the analysis of running shoes is the heel-counter. This is the cuff of the heel at the back of the shoe. It should be deep enough to allow support of the entire heel portion of the foot.

You should check that it's firm enough to provide good support for the heel through the various phases of running. Most good running shoes have a heel-counter made of a polyurethane material. But, there are some shoes which still use cardboard. The way to tell is that the shoes with cardboard are softer when you push your thumb into this part of the shoe. These shoes should be avoided. Cardboard becomes weakened when it gets wet and the support of the heel counter reduced dramatically. This in turn significantly affects the support of the foot during running.

In the heel portion of the shoe, the sole should also be carefully checked. It's very important that there's not excessive wearing of the insole, the outer sole or of the shoe in the region of the heel. This can cause a twisting effect on the heel which can lead to injuries of the ankle joint and the joint just below this. These are important joints in maintaining stability of the foot in twisting and turning manoeuvres.

Finally, the outer sole of the shoe, or the tread, should also be checked. You should make sure that there are adequate groovings in the tread of the outer sole to enable a good grip on a loose surface and also in wet or slushy conditions which may prevail when running on grass.

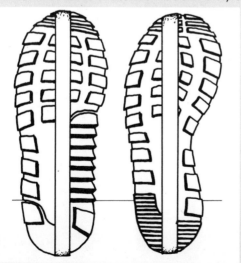

A straight-lasted shoe (left) and a curve-lasted shoe (right).

LITTLE ATHLETICS

COMMON INJURIES

Muscle injuries

Injuries mainly occurring in athletic events, particularly running, are those to muscles and tendons as well as to some joints involving the ligaments and capsules.

One incident of overstress can damage a muscle or tendon.

In short running events such as sprints or middle-distance running, or in jumping and throwing events, one incident of overstress can damage a muscle or tendon. Typically, the muscle or tendon is suddenly stressed beyond its capabilities at one particular instant. This causes some damage to muscle fibres whether they be in the middle portion of the muscle or where the muscle becomes a tendon at the attachment on a bone.

A muscle usually begins at a bone. It then develops into a muscle belly made up of many thousands of muscle fibres. This then tapers down into a muscle tendon junction continuing on as a tendon. It then inserts on to another bone, acting across a joint to enable the movement of portion of a limb. This is, in turn, acted upon by this muscle-tendon unit.

The various areas where damage can occur from an overstress situation are at the origin of the muscle, within the muscle belly itself, at the junction of the muscle and tendon and either within the tendon substance or near its insertion on the bone.

At each of these areas, when overstress occurs, there's damage to the muscle and/or tendon fibres. The athlete immediately experiences pain which can prevent the completion of the activity.

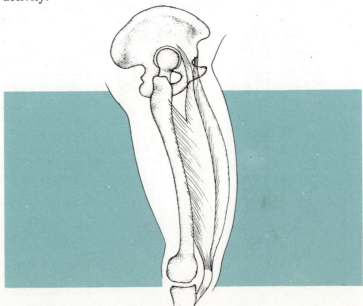

One of the thigh muscles commonly injured from an overstress.

34

LITTLE ATHLETICS

In sprinters and jumpers, this muscle injury commonly occurs in the hamstrings and thigh muscles. But, it occasionally strikes in the calf muscle extending into the Achilles tendon. In middle-distance runners, the injuries mainly involve the legs and again can occur in the hamstring muscles, the calf muscles and the Achilles tendon.

For those who participate in throwing sports, the injuries can occur in the legs together with the possibility of muscle and/or tendon damage in the upper arms. Particularly at risk are the biceps and triceps muscles and also the muscles supporting the shoulder joint.

Immediately a young athlete experiences pain in one of these areas the activity should be stopped and ice applied in the form of an ice pack wrapped in a wet towel over the painful area. The ice pack should be firmly applied with an elasticised bandage for compression.

Apply ice as soon as pain is experienced.

If possible, the injured area should be elevated to help in the reduction of fluid formation whether it be damage to muscles or tendons.

Usually, in young children and adolescents, the muscle or tendon damage is only mild or moderately severe. Pain and irritation to the damaged area will be significantly reduced with the application of ice, compression and elevation over the next 24 to 48 hours. Following this treatment, simple stretching manoeuvres can be started. These will enable the muscles to resume some of their normal activities without allowing excessive contraction of the muscle or the scar tissue. This speeds rehabilitation and also prevents excessive stiffness and contracture.

Simple stretching manoeuvres speed rehabilitation.

If the area of tissue damage is localised, ice massage can be performed for three or four days while doing these stretching manoeuvres. The ice should be held in a towel. Alternatively, use ice which has been frozen in a polystyrene cup with the lip of the cup broken away to expose the ice. The ice can then be directly applied to the skin, massaging in the direction of the muscle fibres to relieve muscle spasm and tightness. This is particularly effective following an exercise program which has considerably stretched the muscle.

There are specific exercises which can be performed to initially stretch the muscle after injury. There are different exercises depending upon the area of the body where the injury has occurred, the nature of the accident and the muscle which has been damaged.

These exercises should be done without resistance or any weights and gradually, within the limits of pain, you should increase the intensity and number of repetitions to stretch and strengthen the muscle-tendon structures.

LITTLE ATHLETICS

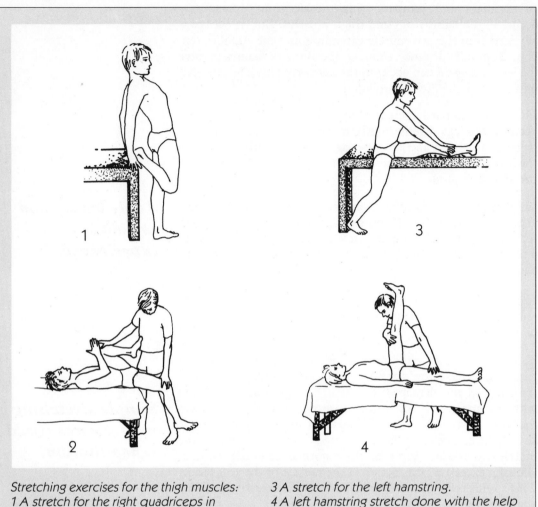

Stretching exercises for the thigh muscles:
1 A stretch for the right quadriceps in upright position.
2 A left hip flexor stretch done with the help of a friend.
3 A stretch for the left hamstring.
4 A left hamstring stretch done with the help of a friend.

Once the young athlete can fully stretch the affected muscle-tendon unit without pain, and has also undergone at least two or three days of intense strengthening exercises, then some training can be resumed. This should specifically involve the previously damaged muscle-tendon unit.

A specific retraining program is very important.

It's very important that the young athlete undergoes a specific retraining program which includes education about how the injury happened. This effectively promotes an understanding of appropriate measures to avoid reinjury.

Always start with an adequate warm-up.

Emphasis should be on an adequate warm-up before training, or competition, which involves not only specific stretching exercises for the previously damaged muscle-tendon unit, but also should include exercises that stretch the commonly used muscle groups for that particular physical activity.

LITTLE ATHLETICS

It may also be advisable to apply ice to the previously injured muscle following training, or after competition, for about 10 to 15 minutes particularly in the two to three weeks after the return to normal training and competition, to again prevent any further accumulation of fluid in this area. This also avoids any spasm or contraction of the muscle-tendon unit.

Apply ice after training or competition.

Preventive measures, such as a proper warm-up, a stretching program, and icing down following intensive physical activities following an injury, are helpful in preventing recurrence of the injury. They also make the athlete aware of how tissues can be injured as well as the best ways to avoid such injuries from occurring.

Iliotibial band

Specific running injuries predominately involve the legs and, in children, the feet, the Achilles tendon and a band of tissue that runs down the outer side of the thigh from the hip towards the outer surface of the knee.

This band of tissue is known as the iliotibial band. It comprises a tendinous substance that has the function of helping the knee in maintaining full extension or straightening. It has an auxiliary significance at the hip joint, particularly in running up or down hills.

This band can become irritated in three common places. The first is near the hip bone. You can feel it on the outer surface of the buttocks at the commencement of the thigh. Here, the band of tissue can rub across the bony prominence at the upper part of the thigh bone. It's here that a bursa, or sac, that helps in the gliding of this band across this bone can become inflamed. A bursitis can form where fluid excessively collects in the sac. The area becomes quite tender when touched or after running some distance.

The band itself can also become irritated in this region. It becomes tender to touch and also tends to become sore soon after the start of running, particularly when trying to run up or down hills.

The second area where this band of tissue can become inflamed is in the mid-portion of the tissue. But, this isn't as common as in the upper aspect of the thigh. Nor is it as common as in the lower aspect where the band runs across the outer aspect of the knee towards its attachment on the tibia — the large bone in the lower leg below the knee.

LITTLE ATHLETICS

The region of the iliotibial band at the knee joint can become irritated when friction occurs, as the band moves slightly across the knee joint when the joint moves from full straightening to full bending. As the band of tissue glides across the bone, it can become irritated and inflamed. This causes pain and irritation when attempting to run and, sometimes, trying to jump.

The best treatment is to avoid the activity.

The best treatment for this condition is to avoid the activity that caused the irritation for a while. If a specific correlation between the injury and running on hills is found, this should also be avoided for about four to six weeks.

Ice massage is also very beneficial for this condition, using the method previously described — an ice block held in a piece of towel or a refrigerated polystyrene cup of ice. Where the specific irritation is localised, the application of ice massage in a rhythmical manner is good for reducing inflammation.

If the inflammation persists, seek medical advice. A mild, oral anti-inflammatory medication is often prescribed to help with the ice massage in reducing the inflammation and scarring in the area of tissue damage.

Once the inflammation and the pain have subsided then gentle stretching can be performed. There are specific exercises for the iliotibial band. They should be performed in groups of three repetitions followed by the application of ice massage.

Jogging can recommence once the athlete is able to fully stretch the iliotibial band without pain and when there's no specific pain at rest. There can be a gradual increase over a two- to three-week period in the running intensity, duration and frequency. But, it's best to avoid hill running until the athlete can run pain-free for a considerable length of time on flat terrain.

LITTLE ATHLETICS

WHEN IS IT SAFE TO GO BACK WITHOUT RISKING REINJURY?

There are four main aspects in any running program:

★ The number of runs each week.
★ The distance or duration of each run.
★ The intensity of the session that is, the speed of the run and whether sprinting or other activities are incorporated.
★ The nature of the terrain, particularly the variation between flat and hilly surfaces.

The reintroduction of the running program after an injury should include the gradual increase of each of these variables one at a time. They should only be increased gradually, one variable at a time, to allow the body to readjust without the risk of a recurrence of an injury or the development of a different one.

Over an extended period, which may be six to eight weeks, I usually recommend that the runner return to jogging, possibly two to three times a week. Keep the distance to maybe a third of the distance of the usual training program. Then, gradually, increase the duration of the run, still running two or three times a week.

Once normal training distance has been reached, the number of runs can be gradually increased to the number performed before the injury. Then introduce changes to the intensity of the runs. Finally introduce variations to the terrain, particularly taking note of the type of injury sustained. For example, if recovering from an iliotibial band injury, you should very slowly reintroduce the child to hill running as the last variable in the resumption of the training program.

Inflammation of the patella tendon

Another common running injury in young runners is the development of inflammation of the patella tendon.

This is a tendon extending from the thigh muscle to surround the kneecap (the patella) to continue on to insert in the front of the tibia (lower leg bone below the knee joint).

Inflammation of this tendon in runners can occur just above the kneecap, just below the kneecap and also at the point of insertion on the tibia.

Again, the cornerstone of treatment is rest and the avoidance of running until the inflammation has subsided. Ice massage should also be applied together with specific stretching exercises for the quadriceps / hamstrings.

Treat this with rest and ice massage.

Stress fractures

Fortunately, stress fractures are not as common in young children and adolescents as they are in adult long-distance runners. But, with the popularity of long-distance running and the dramatic distances that young children have been running over the last two years, there's been an upsurge in the development of stress fractures in the bones of the lower limbs — particularly, the tibia, and the fibula (the two bones of the lower leg) and also some small bones of the foot.

LITTLE ATHLETICS

Prolonged overuse can cause stress fractures.

Stress fractures are usually caused by prolonged overuse. But, on occasions they can be caused by one specific instance of overstress which results in damage to the structure of the bone.

Treatment of stress fractures is usually the same as a normal fracture of the bone — except that, on occasions, the application of a plaster of Paris cast is not required as there's no deformity.

Provided the young athlete avoids excessive stress on that injured part of the body, the main treatment is rest to allow the bone to heal. This usually takes four to six weeks.

DIAGNOSING A STRESS FRACTURE IS DIFFICULT

Sometimes it can be very difficult to make an accurate diagnosis of a stress fracture from an X-ray. The only clinical finding is often an area of diffuse pain in the lower leg.

A specific investigation known as a bone scan is often required. This involves a radioactive dye injected into the vein. Over a period of several hours, the dye circulates through the body and concentrates in areas of calcium deposits or new bone formation.

Where there's a fracture, calcium deposits increase as part of the overall bone healing process. There's an increase in the uptake of dye in such an area which shows up as a 'hot spot' on the scan clearly identifying the position of the stress fracture.

Achilles tendon problems

In the young runner, irritation to the Achilles tendon is not uncommon. Inflammation can result in the lower part of the calf extending to behind the ankle and even down to the insertion of the tendo-Achilles on the back of the heel bone.

This can be caused by excessive use of the calf muscle.

Usually, inflammation in the Achilles tendon occurs as the result of an overuse syndrome. Excessive use of the calf muscle is often the cause.

The treatment should therefore involve rest and ice massage and again specific stretching and strengthening exercises for the calf muscle as shown in the following diagrams.

These exercises should be done regularly, two or three times a day, with three sets of 20 repetitions of each exercise. It's also very important to strengthen the calf muscles before returning to a running program.

Lack of strength causes reinjury.

It's essential with any muscle or tendon injury that the combination of stretching and strengthening exercises be performed in the rehabilitation period. Lack of strength in the muscle is one of the common causes of reinjury to the area when you return to a strenuous activity such as running.

40

LITTLE ATHLETICS

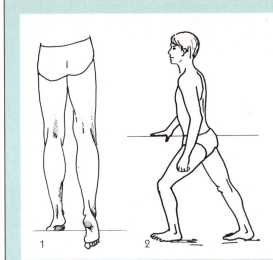

1 *Toe raises for calf muscle strengthening help prevent Achilles tendon injuries.*

2 *Combined calf stretching and Achilles tendon exercise. To complete the exercise reverse the leg position and stretch again.*

Common foot injuries in long-distance running

Finally, I would like to briefly discuss some injuries which can occur in the foot as a result of long-distance running. The most common is inflammation to the band of tissue which runs across the sole of the foot from the front of the heel bone to the bases of all of the toes. Known as the plantar fascia, it's a very important ligament which helps maintain the arches of the foot and prevents the forebones of the foot from spreading out, particularly when taking weight on the foot.

This band of tissue or ligament can become inflamed near its attachment on the front of the heel bone, commonly on the inner side of the foot. But, the inflammation can also occur in the mid-substance of the ligament, usually on the inner surface. On occasions, it can extend to the bases of the toes. This is a common, and quite painful running injury. If the young athlete tries to keep running or engage in other strenuous activities, severe pain can result. Even walking becomes painful.

No attempt should be made to run. Apply ice massage and possibily introduce oral anti-inflammatory medication. If the pain due to inflammation persists, physiotherapy may be necessary in the form of ultrasonic treatment.

If massage doesn't resolve the problem and the inflammation is quite localised, then an injection of cortisone steroid and a long-lasting local anaesthetic may be necessary to specifically reduce the inflammation in this area. Once this has been administered, it's essential that the athlete completely rest the area for one or two days. This may require the use of crutches with a gradual increase of weight bearing over seven to ten days.

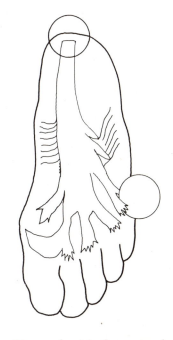

Plantar fascitis. It commonly occurs at the attachment on the heel or near its insertion at the base of the toes. Inflammation can occur on the sole of the foot involving the large supporting ligament.

LITTLE ATHLETICS

Blisters.

Other common foot injuries in runners include the formation of blisters, most frequently over the toes, particularly the inner surface of the big toe and in the outer aspect of the little toe, and also at the back of the heel. This can be caused by an excessive amount of running or ill-fitting shoes.

Blisters should be treated promptly and carefully. Otherwise, infections can cause significant problems in the feet. Not only will they prevent the athlete from returning to running but can also cause much more generalised problems if the infection becomes severe and involves the lymph glands.

Usually, it's best to let the blister burst, or puncture it with a hot needle which has been sterilised in boiling water. Allow the skin overlying the blister to remain unless it's torn away. It's preferable not to cut this skin away because it provides a protective layer over the underlying raw area of new skin.

HELPFUL HINTS

★ Always have a well-organised program. Remember that children in an enclosed area, such as a track and field arena, can be seriously injured if events are not well supervised and not thoughtfully placed so as to minimise the risk of injuries.

★ Always clear the track of any dangerous objects, particularly in running events, because young athletes concentrating intensively on their activities can easily miss any objects lying on the track or in the centre arena.

★ Make sure that the landing pits for the long jump, triple jump and the high jump are adequate and appropriately maintained and supervised by an adult. Be alert to the serious injuries which can occur to the spine, pelvis, and points of the lower limbs due to inadequate landing pits or inappropriately placed rubber pontoons in the high jump area.

★ Shoes are the most important equipment for young athletes engaging in running. Always make sure that:

They are well fitting and have a firm and well-positioned heel counter.

The mid-sole isn't too rigid or too flexible.

The outer sole has a good tread and isn't excessively flared in the region of the heel.

The toe box is of an adequate size to prevent excessive rubbing of the toes which could cause blisters.

★ With running, an adequate warm-up is a must and should include stretching exercises particularly for muscles in the lower limbs, such as the calf, thigh and hamstrings.

★ Common injuries in Little Athletics are to muscles and tendons, caused by one overstress incident, particularly in sprinting, jumping or throwing. This commonly involves the muscles and tendons of the lower limbs. Treatment should include ice massage, rest and avoidance of the activities which caused the problems.

★ Once the pain caused by any inflammation has subsided, immediately introduce specific strengthening and stretching exercises. This should involve not only the muscle and tendon unit, but also other associated muscles in the specific area of the injured part of the body.

★ Children and young adolescents are not little adults. They cannot be expected to perform the same activities at the same intensity as adults. Thus, excessive long-distance running is fraught with danger and can cause serious problems which affect the growth and development of the child.

Football: Australian Rules, Rugby and Soccer

4

PREVENTION

Before discussing the most common injuries let's focus attention on prevention — the most important aspect of all, be it football or any other type of sport.

To assess and evaluate appropriate preventive measures, first carefully look at the arena or surface on which the game is to be played. This includes surrounding fences, goal posts and other facilities required for participation in the game. Also, check any specific equipment that each individual player requires — boots, shinguards and other protective equipment. Be aware of the players themselves. Pay close attention to their fitness level and understanding of the rules of the game. Don't overlook the referees, umpires and officials who have the arduous task of controlling the game.

The playing area

Because our climate is so good, even in winter, most football games are played outdoors except for the recent development of indoor soccer. It's essential that someone carefully check the playing surface before the game starts.

You should look for any protruding objects on the ground which can cause serious injury if a player fell on them. Don't forget underground sprinkler systems which may not be adequately covered. The ground surface should be evenly grassed. Although it's difficult in the summer months, large areas of clay or dirt without an even cover of grass can cause serious abrasions and damage when players fall or twist on to such a surface at high speed.

The ground surface should be evenly grassed.

It's also very important that the boundary line be well away from any fence or other fixed object which may be close to the ground. I believe that about two metres (at least six feet) should be allowed between a boundary and any fence so that players can avoid serious injury if they were to run into the fence or be pushed out of the field by an opposing player.

FOOTBALL

Goal posts should be well padded.

Goal posts should be well padded. Many young players have been seriously injured when running into such uprights at high speed. These include the uprights for soccer. The risk of serious injuries can easily be minimised and even avoided altogether.

Protective equipment

In the codes of football played in Australia, there's very little protective equipment used, except for the use of shoulder pads by rugby players. These should be checked regularly to make sure they are in good order and that they are the right size for the player's age and build. More harm can occur when a player is wearing protective equipment which is too large or too small.

Padded knee bandages are helpful.

Padded knee bandages are helpful for young players troubled by soreness on the front of their knees. This particularly happens in the early part of the season when the weather is warm and the ground is hard. The wearing of such knee and elbow braces can help prevent any further damage to the knee or elbow joints.

Check those boots

Probably, the most important item of equipment of all for football players are boots. They should be a good fitting pair checked regularly to make sure they are not too small or too large. The stops, or studs, should be of the appropriate size. Certainly don't have any sharp or protruding nails or sharp pieces of nylon which can inflict considerable damage to the skin and soft tissues if applied vigorously to an opponent either intentionally or by accident.

Boots should be checked regularly.

A major problem with boots, particularly with young footballers, is that the boots marketed in Australia are low-cut types which don't provide enough ankle support. These are the boots worn by professional footballers and are therefore easily marketed by the major companies to aspiring younger players. Unbeknown to the majority of young footballers, the professional footballers have their ankles strapped with non-elastic tape which is quite rigid. This precaution is taken when training as well as playing. Although the professional footballers prefer the low-cut boots for mobility and speed, the added protection of strapping helps minimise twisting injuries which can occur to the ankle joint.

Encourage under-16 players to wear high-cut boots.

Because the young footballer usually doesn't have the luxury of such protection, I strongly believe that footballers under the age of 16 should be encouraged to wear higher cut boots to avoid the risk of injury.

FOOTBALL

There's much hard evidence that high-cut boots don't impede mobility or speed of movement. But they certainly give the player added protection from the frequent twisting and turning of the ankle and foot in all codes of football.

The real problem parents have is that the boots are not readily available. They also have to convince their young budding footballers that low-cut boots won't somehow transform them into superstars.

The importance of adequate pre-season training

It's very important when players are participating in a contact sport that an appropriate time in the pre-season is given to reaching and maintaining a minimum fitness level. This enables the individual players to attain a skill level relevant to their particular code of football. Players can then perform in a game situation with an enhanced ability to withstand the gruelling stresses applied to the body throughout the game.

This thorough pre-season preparation produces muscles which are flexible and strong as well as supporting joints which are aware of what is required of them for a particular movement. They are better able to withstand the intensity of forces and stresses applied to them during decisive moments of the game.

Good pre-season training produces strong, flexible muscles.

Know the rules

Don't just think you know the rules, make certain you do. Significant injury reduction also comes from knowing, and applying, the rules of the particular code. This is a close second to practising self-help injury prevention by achieving, and maintaining, a high level of fitness and improved strength and flexibility.

Make certain you know the rules.

A complete understanding of the rules of the particular code being played will often prevent the unnecessary, injury-charged risk situations of conflict between players.

Other preventive factors are the umpires and officials. It's imperative that these officials know and understand the rules of the particular code and consistently apply them.

Less ignorance by all involved means avoiding unnecessary confusion and conflict between players with fewer injuries likely. Injuries can, however, only be reduced, never eliminated. The very nature of football, and other vigorous contact sports, inevitably means players being injured.

FOOTBALL

INFECTION IS THE BIG DANGER. NEVER TAKE CHANCES.

As football is mostly played outdoors, when a player hits the ground hard injuries occur to the skin, frequently in the form of cuts and abrasions.

Unless the cut is substantial, these injuries often don't become evident until the end of the game when the player notices that an area of skin around the knee or elbow joint has been damaged — usually an abrasion with some minor cuts.

Avoiding infection is the most important factor in treating these injuries. The best policy is always prevention.

A scrubbing brush became the most feared object by many of the players when I was the club doctor with the Prahran Football Club in the Victorian Football Association. It was the most frequently used part of my medical equipment.

Once I had established who had developed an abrasion to the skin and to what region of the body, I made a frequent journey into the shower room with my scrubbing brush. Despite howls of protest and unprintable exclamations by the players about the cleanliness of the wound, the vigorous application of the scrubbing brush to the injury was a very efficient way of removing dirt and debris from the wound. It also helped stimulate the blood supply to the region. Once the player had completed his shower, the application of a clean dressing was necessary.

I'm pleased to say that this simple and direct method prevented secondary infection in 99.99 per cent of cases, to the delight of the coach. There's nothing more frustrating to a club than a key player missing several games because of a secondary infection of a skin abrasion.

Clearly, if a player has a large cut which doesn't appear to close easily with the application of sticking plaster or bandage, then prompt medical treatment is necessary to adequately close the wound to promote good healing and minimal scar formation.

Depending on the size and position of the wound, it's not unusual to allow a player to resume training within a few days. But, if there is any concern about the wound, I would keep the player out until the stitches have been removed.

FOOTBALL

COMMON INJURIES
Muscle injuries

In all codes of football and contact sports, direct force applied to the body can result in bruising to the soft tissues beneath the skin and, more importantly, to the muscles which lie just deep enough in the soft tissues.

This direct force results in damage to the muscle tissue which is known as a haematoma — a bleeding within the muscle due to damage of the muscle fibres and the small blood vessels within the tissues.

Clearly, in soccer, these injuries usually occur to the legs from the hips down. But, in rugby and Australian rules football, direct injuries can occur to any part of the body, particularly the shoulders and the upper arms as well as the thighs and the hips. The extent, or size of the injury, is directly related to the amount of damaged muscle tissue.

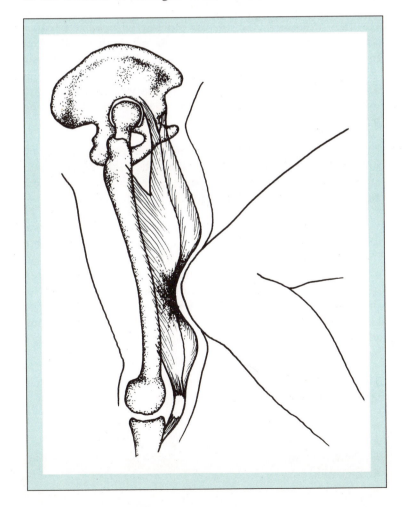

Damage to the thigh muscle usually occurs from a direct blow by an opponent. The damaged muscle usually bleeds forming a haematoma.

FOOTBALL

A muscle strain is also damage to the muscle tissue which results in bleeding and swelling. However, this happens not because of an external force, but rather from the tearing of the muscle fibres when excessive internal forces are applied to the muscle.

Either way, the effect of damage to the muscle tissue is the same. Therefore, the same treatment is used for both a muscle contusion caused by an external force and a muscle strain due to an internal force.

Before describing how to treat a muscle tissue injury, I would like to give you an example of how not to treat such an injury. Hopefully, this will reinforce the advice for appropriate treatment.

Again, when I was the club doctor at Prahran Football Club, I was attending training on a Tuesday night when a father came in concerned about how slowly a wound his son had sustained the previous Saturday was healing.

He then brought in the 14-year-old boy who walked with a noticeable limp. He described how his left thigh had been hit by an opponent's knee and that the leg had quickly become swollen. The local trainer had told him to go home that night and have a hot bath. The next day, he was advised to run some laps of the oval in an attempt to stretch the muscle and 'run out' the injury.

I then asked the young boy to remove his trousers. It was no surprise to see an extremely swollen left thigh. It was about eight centimetres larger in circumference than the right thigh and was extremely tender to touch.

I estimate that he had bled two to three litres of blood into that left thigh. In fact, the fluid was now moving down into the region of his left knee and also down into the left calf muscle. Without the right treatment there would have been further bleeding into the thigh and possibly calcification of the haematoma which is known as 'myositis ossificans'. Unfortunately, this young boy had been given the wrong advice and had applied all the wrong principles of treating a muscle or soft tissue injury.

The cornerstone of treatment for soft tissue bruising, muscle bruising or tearing is RICE:

- ★ Rest
- ★ Ice
- ★ Compression
- ★ Elevation

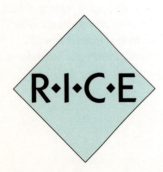

FOOTBALL

With the simple application of these four basic principles of initial treatment for soft tissue injuries, you can avoid serious complications which could result in permanent damage. (The RICE treatment is explained on page 16.)

Once the pain and swelling have subsided, gentle exercise can be commenced within the limitations of pain that is, if it's too painful to stretch the muscle any further, then the exercising should be restricted to the range of movement that can be tolerated. Increase the exercises gradually until a full range of movement is possible. Only then can the player resume more strenuous activities like running, twisting, stretching and eventually participation in the full training program.

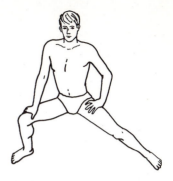

Left thigh adductor stretching exercise. To complete the exercise reverse the leg position and stretch again.

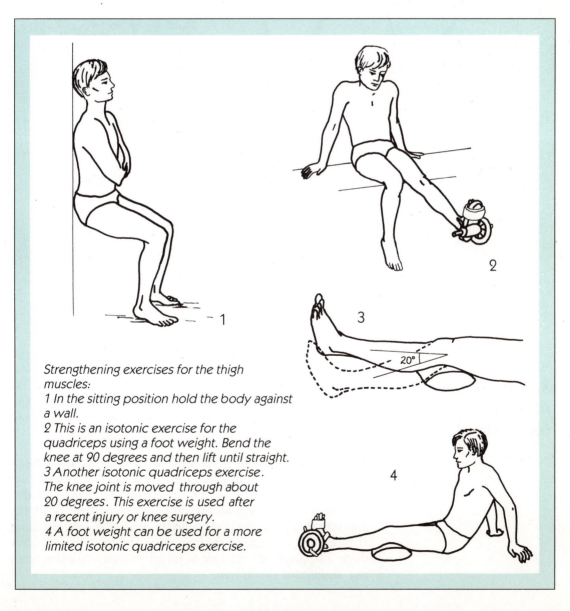

Strengthening exercises for the thigh muscles:
1 In the sitting position hold the body against a wall.
2 This is an isotonic exercise for the quadriceps using a foot weight. Bend the knee at 90 degrees and then lift until straight.
3 Another isotonic quadriceps exercise. The knee joint is moved through about 20 degrees. This exercise is used after a recent injury or knee surgery.
4 A foot weight can be used for a more limited isotonic quadriceps exercise.

JOINT INJURIES

Joint injuries are quite common in all three codes of football. In soccer, they usually involve the ankle and knee joints as well as hand injuries from contact with the ball. In rugby and Australian rules football, joint injury commonly involves the hands and the shoulder girdle, the knee and the ankle joints. With hand injuries, full or partial dislocations of the small joints of the fingers are quite common.

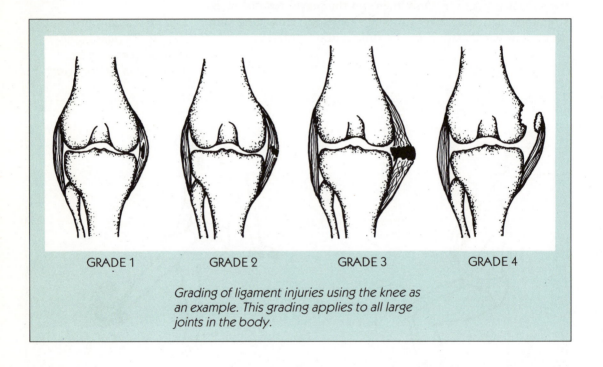

GRADE 1   GRADE 2   GRADE 3   GRADE 4

Grading of ligament injuries using the knee as an example. This grading applies to all large joints in the body.

Finger dislocations

Splint a dislocated finger immediately.

No matter how urgent the demands of the game, dislocation of the small joint in the finger should mean immediate splinting. It's a simple matter to strap the affected finger to one either side of it. This provides an excellent splint.

The player should then be sent to an appropriate medical facility for an X-ray to make sure there isn't any significant damage to the joint or to the accompanying bone. Usually, there won't be any significant joint or bone damage. With the application of ice and appropriate splinting, the swelling reduces and movement resumes over the next two to three days. The player is then able to return to competition without any significant disruption.

FOOTBALL

However, I always advise that they continue strapping the injured finger to the accompanying one. This allows full movement in the affected joint. Also, the strapping should be done at every training session and during competition for the next two to three weeks.

Shoulder girdle injuries

All injuries to the shoulder girdle are potentially serious. In rugby and Australian rules football, injuries to the shoulder girdle usually occur in the form of a dislocation to the shoulder joint. This often happens when the arm is forced backwards when tackling a player, or when landing awkwardly.

All shoulder girdle injuries are potentially serious.

If the player appears distressed and holds the arm in a protective manner against the side of the body it's possible they have injured the shoulder girdle. Carefully observe the shoulder girdle to see if it looks more square than usual. The square appearance is because the ball of the upper arm bone has been displaced out of the joint socket. It's been forced towards the front of the joint, and also downwards, distorting the normal rounded appearance of the shoulder girdle.

Once this has happened, it's imperative that the player be transported to a medical facility for reduction of the dislocation. During this transportation, I strongly advise that the player be allowed to hold the arm in whatever position he or she feels comfortable with. No attempt should be made to move the arm into what the player or anyone else thinks is a more natural position. Significant pain and also muscle spasm would be likely as the body's natural defences signal the inadvisability of the arm being moved in any further direction which could cause damage to the shoulder joint.

The further treatment and rehabilitation of such an injury should be co-ordinated by a doctor and a physiotherapist before contemplating any return to training or competition.

Treatment and rehabilitation should be under medical supervision.

Another injury, which can occur in the shoulder girdle, particularly in rugby, is damage to the acromioclavicular joint. This is a small joint in the upper aspect of the shoulder girdle between the collar bone and the acromium (at the top of the shoulder).

These injuries usually result from direct contact to the shoulder girdle. In rugby, this usually occurs in the formation of the scrum.

FOOTBALL

The more minor injuries to the acromioclavicular joint can be treated with the application of ice and rest for the first 24 to 48 hours. Alternatively, by the general reduction of movement of the arm as well as the use of oral anti-inflammatory medication such as Feldene, Voltaren or Naprosyn.

The more significant injuries to this joint may require prolonged periods of rest and rehabilitation with physiotherapy treatment, utilising electrotherapy and specific strengthening exercises for the supporting muscles.

The dreaded knee joint injuries

In all codes of football, the injury that the player fears most is an injury to the knee joint. There are a variety of injuries which can occur to the knee joint.

Minor injuries usually involve damage to the meniscus.

Fortunately, the less severe injuries usually occur more often than the severe ones. The minor injuries usually involve damage to the meniscus. There are two compartments in the knee joint — the medial (inner compartment) and the lateral (the outer compartment). Each compartment has a meniscus. This cartilaginous disc can be torn, particularly when a player twists or turns suddenly on his or her leg.

This typically happens when the leg is fixed, for example, stuck in mud, or when an opponent is standing on a player's foot. Such a rotation of the knee joint can result in a torn meniscus, which is usually accompanied by some damage to the capsule surrounding the knee joint. Damage can also occur to the ligamentous structures supporting the joint.

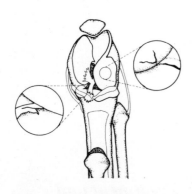

The inside of the knee can be easily damaged in sports involving twisting or pivoting. The damage is usually to either the meniscus on the left or to the cartilage lining of the joint as shown on the right.

The ligaments supporting the knee joint are divided into two groups. The ligaments within the joint itself are known as the anterior and the posterior cruciate ligaments. The ligaments outside the joint capsule are known as the medial and lateral collateral ligaments.

If the knee joint becomes swollen within the first four hours following injury, it must be assumed that bleeding has occurred within the joint. This may be caused by a fracture to one of the bones within the joint, damage to one of the internal ligaments or the tearing of the meniscus.

If this rapid swelling occurs, immediate medical treatment should be started. If there are delays in providing such treatment, then the application of RICE is strongly recommended until a doctor sees the player.

FOOTBALL

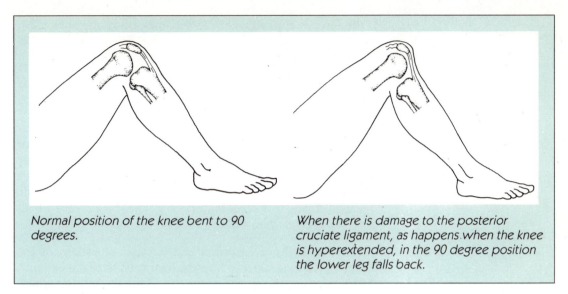

Normal position of the knee bent to 90 degrees.

When there is damage to the posterior cruciate ligament, as happens when the knee is hyperextended, in the 90 degree position the lower leg falls back.

However, if the swelling in the knee joint occurs slowly, that is, over a 24-hour period, it's usually due to irritation of the synovium — the inner lining under the capsule joint. Such irritation causes an increase of the fluid normally produced by the synovium. This in turn results in a swelling within the joint.

The problem isn't as urgent as that with rapid swelling in the joint, but the application of RICE is vitally important. If an improvement doesn't occur within two to three days, then I would recommend you seek medical advice about the best management of the injury.

A major advance in recent years is that doctors can now see the internal aspects of a joint using a procedure known as arthroscopy. An arthroscope is a tiny telescope with a light source. Not only the knee joint, but also the shoulder, ankle and the elbow joints can be seen using this procedure.

A small hole is made and an arthroscope is inserted in the joint and, through other small holes into the joint, instruments can be inserted and appropriate procedures performed within the joint.

This avoids the need to make a large incision for investigative procedures. Hospitalisation time has been greatly reduced and the post-operative rehabilitation process speeded. A more significant intervention may be called for with a more major injury to the external or internal ligaments supporting the knee joint.

Injuries to the external ligaments of the knee joint usually happen when a player is twisting, or pivoting, and collides with an opponent. The sideways force to the knee joint, applied to the outside of the knee joint, stresses the inner ligaments known as the medial collateral ligament.

FOOTBALL

If the force is applied from the inside aspect of the knee joint, the damage occurs to the outer ligament, known as the lateral collateral ligament.

Because it's far more common for the force to be applied from the outside, a medial collateral ligament injury is the more usual of the two complaints.

A sports medicine doctor typically sees various types, or stages of injury, from the more minor resulting from damage to a small portion of the ligament fibres, to a moderate injury which typically involves damage to 40 to 60 per cent of the ligament fibres, to a severe injury or a type three injury which involves greater than 60 per cent of the ligament fibres.

Clearly, with the progression of the type, or extent, of the injury to the external and internal ligaments to the knee joint, this determines the extent of the instability to the joint which becomes evident upon examination of the joint.

In a significant injury to the knee joint involving the ligaments it's also quite common to see damage to the capsule and nerve endings which supply information to the brain about the function of the knee joint.

An example comes to mind of a football match when a player received a significant injury to his right knee joint and was taken from the ground. My initial examination showed he had completely disrupted his anterior cruciate ligament and his medial and lateral collateral ligaments. However, he had felt no pain, and in fact, because it was a grand final, was quite keen to return. He actually tried to stand and take a few steps before the knee completely collapsed from under him. It was only then that he realised the full seriousness of the injury to his knee joint. Within half an hour, the knee was swollen and quite painful. But in those initial few minutes following the injury, he was quite oblivious to how serious the injury was. He had felt no pain because of the damage which had occurred to the nerve receptors within the capsule of the joint itself.

THE VALUE OF NON-STRETCH TAPES

Non-stretch tapes applied to joints may do two things. Firstly, a small amount of mechanical support may be given to ligamentous structures. Secondly, proprioception (sensory response) may be enhanced. Some United States studies have suggested that ankle strapping reduces the rate of being injured again within a few months. It's suggested that the main protective mechanism is enhancing the proprioceptive responses and controlling the way the foot is placed. (See page 14 for a full discussion.)

FOOTBALL

THE RISK OF SERIOUS INJURIES

Unfortunately, the vigorous nature of contact sports such as football, carries the risk of serious injury to the head, the eyes, and also to internal organs such as the lungs, the spleen and kidneys because of direct forces being applied to the chest and abdomen.

Head injuries

Closed head injuries (no open cuts but possible internal bruising or bleeding) are not uncommon in football. They can result in brief unconsciousness. It's therefore important when assessing closed head injuries to inquire if there's been any loss of consciousness, or if the player feels dazed and confused. Their level of arousal should be clearly established and also whether there's been any short-term memory loss.

Ask simple questions such as:
★ What's your name?
★ What position were you playing in?
★ Which direction were you kicking?
★ What stage was the game at when you were injured?
★ What's the score?

All these questions are very important in establishing whether he or she has sustained a head injury. If there's concern about a possible head injury, always err on the side of caution, particularly with young players. Immediately remove them from the ground to avoid the risk of further injury and more serious complications.

Always err on the side of caution.

If the player continues to have symptoms such as sleepiness, difficulty in arousal, the development of nausea and vomiting, then prompt evaluation and observation for at least four to six hours is a must.

Remove an injured player from the ground immediately.

My rule when dealing with players involved in contact sports, is to ban them from playing contact sports for two to three weeks if they have sustained a closed head injury. This applies even if temporary loss of consciousness hasn't occurred. This safeguard of insisting on a rest period particularly applies to children or young adolescents. Never take risks with possible head injuries.

Never take risks with head injuries.

The danger of spinal injuries in rugby

Rugby, because of the nature of the sport, involves the risk of spinal injuries, particularly in the scrum when players are in position applying a force straight down the spine. Either hitting the head directly or by hitting the shoulder, shock force is applied down the spine.

FOOTBALL

The danger of spinal injuries was recently highlighted in the United States in gridiron when they had to make a rule change on a tackle known as 'spearing'. A player tackling an opponent would put his head down (and he had a helmet on to protect him) and actually dive like a spear to hit his opponent. While they might not get too bad a head injury because they were wearing a helmet, the force could travel straight down the head, where the helmet finished, to where the cervical spine created a nice fulcrum to snap about C6 or C7 and result in the victim being a low quadriplegic.

There only has to be one or two of these injuries in high school football, with subsequent court cases and big damages awards, and the incentive for sports administrators to reduce such injury risks becomes obvious. Such injuries can happen all too easily, particularly in rugby where a player is down in a position where the forces generated are like being hit by a small car at 60 kilometres per hour.

While a problem with all football codes, rugby has a specific problem in the way players tackle and throw an opponent to the ground.

Strict application of the rules is essential.

The important point for children's sport is that there must be a very strict application and understanding of the rules by the referee and the administrators. This understanding also applies to parents so they don't start accusing the referee of not having good reasons for holding up a game. I believe there should be very strict rules about the scrum, how it's formed and the age of the players.

The sport poses particular dangers to the cervical spine or the neck because an injury to this area can cause quite catastrophic damage to the spinal cord resulting in quadriplegia, very high paraplegia or even death.

A suspected spinal injury requires urgent medical attention. Such an injury should be suspected if a patient has numbness or pins and needles or complains of this below the level of the region where the injury is suspected. For example, below the neck or the shoulders or in the arms, hands, abdomen or legs. If they're unable to move muscle groups in their arms or legs, or if they have pain in the spinal region then also suspect a spinal cord injury. A spinal cord injury should also be suspected if they have received a severe blow to the forehead or a whiplash-type movement of their neck.

FOOTBALL

The important point is that anyone suspected of having sustained a spinal injury should not be moved unless under medical supervision. That's the absolute bottom line in using commonsense caution. It should be in capitals and underlined in your mind. Even minor fractures of the vertebrae can lead to quadriplegia or paraplegia if faulty moving techniques produce dislocation of the fractured vertebrae.

> **STOP**
> *Do not move a player with a suspected spinal injury.*

Chest injuries to footballers

Injuries to the chest due to direct forces being applied are not uncommon in Australian rules football and rugby. Fractured ribs can occur which may result in damage to lung and pleural tissues and also there is the possibility of damage to the spleen which lies under the left diaphragm in the upper part of the left side of the abdomen.

Sometimes, it's difficult to assess whether the player has developed a serious internal injury. This is where it's important, if you're a trainer or coach, that you know your players — particularly how they respond to injuries. This will sharpen your perception of whether or not they are seriously injured.

The example comes to mind of my first match as the club doctor with the Prahran Football Club. During the first quarter, George Stone, who was a very determined player, was involved in a collision with an opponent. George felt some pain on the left side of his chest and upper abdomen. I examined him during the quarter time interval. During the examination, he was mildly tender over the left mid to lower rib cage. But he was breathing reasonably well with only mild to moderate discomfort. I asked him whether he was able to keep playing. He replied that he was fine and that he wanted to go back the next quarter. By the time I had left the ground and had walked up the stairs to the coach's box, the game had started. When the ball had been bounced, George Stone attempted to run towards it. He immediately stopped and bent over.

When I saw this, I asked the coach was this normal practice for this particular player. He said this was most unusual, so I immediately got George off the field. An examination with a stethoscope indicated little, or no, air was entering the left side of his chest. I immediately sent him by car to the local hospital where an X-ray revealed two fractured ribs and a collapsed left lung.

He was in hospital for three days. Within three weeks he had resumed training and played five weeks after the injury.

FOOTBALL

THE FIRST FEW HOURS ARE VITAL

I cannot stress enough the importance of erring on the side of being cautious when dealing with any injury in contact sports, whether it involves a joint, the head, the eyes or internal organs.

Commonsense and basic first aid can aid in recovery.

The first few hours following the injury are vital in obtaining the appropriate treatment to avoid serious complications. Simple commonsense and basic first aid principles, particularly when dealing with soft tissue or muscle injuries, or injuries to a joint, can significantly aid in the recovery from such an injury and in preventing more significant secondary problems from occurring.

If not dealt with properly, an injury could delay the player's return to normal competition and also possibly permanently restrict the function of the injured part of the body. Functional disability could result in restricting even the normal activities of daily living. So, proceed with caution.

HELPFUL HINTS

PREVENTION

★ Make sure that the playing arena is always clear of any dangerous objects such as a protruding sprinkler system. Also make sure that the goal posts are padded and that the boundary line is well away from any fences or cars parked around the arena.

★ Make sure that the players' equipment is well fitting and in good working order. This includes boots, making sure that there are no sharp nails protruding from the stops and also that nylon studs haven't worn down excessively.

★ Be sure that each player is flexible and has had a good pre-season training session to develop muscle strength, joint mobility and particularly the acquisition of skills.

★ It's very important that the players, club officials, umpires and referees understand all the rules governing the game. This will go a long way towards reducing injury risks.

TREATMENT

★ Always err on the side of caution when dealing with head injuries, chest or abdominal injuries as well as injuries to joints and muscles. When in doubt, seek medical advice.

★ The first four to six hours following any injury are vital for getting the maximum effects of any treatment and also for minimising any serious complications.

★ The cornerstone of any treatment in contact sports for injuries involving muscles, ligaments or joints is RICE.

Bat and Ball Sports: Cricket, Baseball, Softball and Field Hockey

5

There's always a risk when children play sports that involve the use of hard balls. However, serious injuries can be minimised with the appropriate protective equipment and a keen understanding of the rules.

In sports like cricket, baseball and field hockey, the hardness of the ball should be reduced with younger children, allowing them to enjoy participation in such sports without the fear of being hurt. Rather than have young children play these sports with a lot of protective equipment, it would be preferable to use softer balls, particularly in cricket and baseball, until they get older and participate at a more competitive level. Fortunately, in softball the ball is relatively soft. Even so, if thrown at a high speed, it can cause considerable bruising and damage to skin and underlying soft tissues. It can even cause broken bones if it hits an extremity such as an extended finger.

Use softer balls.

In field hockey the strict application of the rules not allowing players to swing their sticks above shoulder height is very important in minimising serious facial or head injuries which can occur in the more heated moments of the game.

It's also important in cricket, baseball and softball that there's strict adherence to the rules to avoid particularly serious facial or head injuries if the ball is intentionally thrown towards an opponent. Many nasty injuries can result, particularly to the face and eyes.

PROTECTIVE EQUIPMENT

Gloves, shinpads and groin protectors for boys are very important as they protect areas of the body that can be damaged even by a ball thrown at speed. A cricket or baseball striking a batter's fingers can damage the soft tissues and bones. So choose the right sort of gloves — right-handed gloves for those who bat right-handed or else proper left-handed gloves.

It is important to choose the right sort of gloves.

59

In field hockey shinpads are very helpful in minimising injuries which can occur to the lower leg either from the ball or from an indiscriminate swing from an opponent's stick.

Groin protectors are appropriate in cricket, baseball, softball and field hockey because an ill-directed ball can cause considerable damage. For adolescent girls, special bras with breast protection may also help prevent serious bruising, particularly when batting in cricket, softball and baseball.

Helmets

Visors can restrict a young player's ability to see.

I don't believe young children should wear the specialised helmets and face protectors that older adolescents and adults wear for senior cricket. Visors across the face can actually restrict rather than improve a young player's ability to see the ball.

If a protective helmet is to be worn by older children playing cricket or baseball for batting and close-in fielding, I recommend a helmet without a faceguard or visor. Use a firm helmet similar to that worn by baseballers which particularly protects the temple area.

Using softer balls and avoiding short-pitched deliveries which rise up towards the head are practical ways of avoiding serious face or head injuries.

Footwear

High-cut boots reduce the risk of ankle sprains.

Proper footwear is vital in reducing skin injuries involving the sole of the feet and around the toes. High-cut boots for cricketers, particularly bowlers, greatly reduce the risk of ankle sprains. For fast bowlers, or those who are on their feet and are bowling for long periods, shock-absorbing insoles of Sorbathane (a trademark name) can significantly reduce stress placed on the joints of the lumbar spine, therefore reducing the incidence of spinal stress fractures.

Make sure it fits

Parents often overlook the fact that if the equipment isn't the right size, or is otherwise uncomfortable, players won't use it. Lack of thought in selecting the right equipment is a recipe for disaster as serious injuries can occur if the basic items of safety gear are not worn.

BAT AND BALL SPORTS

PREVENTION

As all bat and ball sports are usually played on an outdoor field, it's important to carefully check the field and remove any objects thoughtlessly left lying about.

Make sure that the boundary lines are drawn and clearly mark the field edges. Boundaries should always be well away from large immovable objects such as fences, posts or sheds, that players can run into when they are intently watching the ball, or an opponent coming at them. Simply following these rules will help to avoid serious bone and internal injuries.

INJURIES

When the ball — or on occasions the bat or stick — hits a player, it most commonly bruises the skin and the underlying soft tissues without actually breaking the skin. More severe bruising may be caused to the underlying muscle. Apply ice to the affected area as soon as possible, using either crushed ice in a wet towel or one of the commercially available ice packs. When applying these commercial ice packs, place a wet towel between the ice pack and the skin to avoid burning.

It's vital to reduce the initial swelling due to any bleeding under the skin if small blood vessels have been damaged or, later on, swelling due to fluid as an inflammatory response to the injury sustained to the soft tissues.

Ice should, therefore, be applied for about 20 minutes every three or four hours over the next 24 hours. This will significantly reduce swelling and any extensive scarring that may occur to the soft tissue because of the build-up of fluid.

Apply ice as soon as possible to a bruise.

Rest the injured area, particularly for the first 24 to 48 hours. This promotes maximum healing as blood is diverted from the active muscles to the area where the injury has occurred.

If an extremity such as a finger has been damaged, apply a splint with a bandage to rest the area for a few days. Where the bruising involves deeper structures, particularly the muscles, then the period of splinting may have to be prolonged and also the application of ice may be extended for two or three days.

It's important to resume movement of the injured area as soon as the pain has been reduced to avoid stiffness of the joints above or below the damaged area. Begin movement slowly, within the limitations of pain, with a slow, stretching program for the injured muscles.

BAT AND BALL SPORTS

Damage to bones and joints

Sometimes it's very difficult to establish whether an underlying bone has also been damaged. This is particularly true of the forearm and hand, where there's very little soft tissue padding between skin and bone.

If there's an obvious deformity in the alignment of the bones and the injury is not in an area where there's a joint, assume there's a broken bone. Splint the area and transport the player to a hospital or medical facility for X-rays.

Immediately reduce a dislocation or immobilise a fracture.

If the damaged area involves a joint and there's a deformity when compared with the corresponding body part on the other side, the injury may be either a fracture or a dislocation of the joint. Reduction of a dislocation or immobilisation of a fracture must be done immediately and the player should be promptly sent for X-rays and other appropriate medical treatment.

Sometimes a ball, bat or stick may hit a forearm and cause what appears to be a contusion. However, as the forearm bones can be very close to the skin, it may be a fracture even though there's no sign of deformity. So be alert and err on the side of caution.

'Spot-on' diagnosis

I well remember making a wrong diagnosis when I was medical officer for the Victorian Cricket Team. It was late on the second day of a match being played at the Junction Oval between Victoria and Western Australia. Victoria was in trouble, having lost two early wickets when Graham Yallop was struck a nasty blow on the right forearm from a short-pitched delivery from Mick Malone.

Before I went out to the crease to inspect Yallop's injury, the Victorian team captain, John Scholes emphasised the importance of Yallop continuing to bat. Yallop was in considerable pain when I examined his arm. There was a tender area over the mid-portion of the forearm but, no obvious deformity.

BAT AND BALL SPORTS

I told him that he had probably just sustained some deep bruising and advised him to keep batting. As I returned to the dressing room, he drove the next ball from Malone for four runs, and I felt quite pleased with my decision to keep him batting.

At the end of the day's play, 40 minutes later, I examined Yallop's arm again in the dressing room. Because it was quite tender over the ulna, which is one of the forearm bones, I decided he should have an X-ray just to make sure it wasn't broken.

To my surprise, there was a fracture through the ulna which was undisplaced, and Yallop had to have his right arm immobilised in a plaster cast for the next six weeks. I was henceforth nicknamed 'spot on', a facetious reference to my accuracy in diagnosing this injury.

Rotator cuff lesion

In cricket, softball and baseball, throwing or bowling can place excessive stress on the shoulder and elbow joints. This action, although varying from a bent arm throw in baseball to bowling overarm with a straight arm in cricket and throwing the ball underarm when pitching in softball, can cause stress resulting in damage to the capsules and ligaments which support the joints.

Also, the outfielders and infielders in these three sports can also sustain injuries to the elbow and shoulder joints particularly when attempting to throw the ball either a long distance or very quickly back to another fieldsman.

A common shoulder joint injury occurs in the tendons of those muscles that perform rotation movements. This is known as a rotator cuff lesion. This may either be a tearing of the combined tendon of four small muscles at the shoulder joint or irritation of one or more of the tendons, also known as tenosynovitis (the well-known complaint of Repetitive Strain Injury, or RSI, sufferers).

Rotator cuff lesion can result in thickening of the tendon. Difficulty then arises when the tendon has to move through a small bony canal in the shoulder joint when rotating the arm or lifting it up from the side.

The best treatment should involve rest from the sporting activity until pain and irritation subside. Ice should also be applied to the shoulder joint. Analgesics and anti-inflammatory medication may be needed to ease excessive discomfort. Seek medical advice if the irritation in the shoulder girdle doesn't resolve itself over 10 to 14 days with rest and ice.

The best treatment involves rest.

BAT AND BALL SPORTS

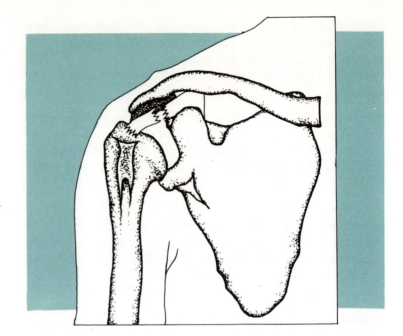

Rotator cuff lesions. Either inflammation or tearing can occur in this area of the shoulder.

Most cases of elbow pain can be successfully treated with rest.

Irritation to the elbow joint is a common injury for fielders who throw the ball fairly regularly or very hard, and also with baseball pitchers.

The many different problems that can occur at the elbow include strains of the muscles around the elbow joint, inflammation of the medial or lateral epicondyle, fractures of the elbow joint bones, and the development of spurs and degenerative changes in the joint.

In the 1960s, the development of the Pee Wee League in the United States lead to an epidemic of elbow problems. Stress placed on the elbow by the pitching action has since been found to be the cause of multiple pathological conditons collectively known as 'Little Leaguer's Elbow'.

A player with Little Leaguer's Elbow usually complains of pain and, as a result, may be unable to throw. The pain can be generalised around the elbow joint because of the different areas that can be irritated. There may be some swelling, and prolonged activity can produce stiffness in the joint which decreases the range of movement.

Most cases of elbow pain caused by excessive pitching can be successfully treated by rest and, if necessary, by splinting. Anti-inflammatory medication and the application of ice may also be necessary in more resistant cases.

However, prevention is the best treatment of all. The Little League has rules that limit the amount a child may pitch during a game. And, in the very young baseball league, known here also as the Pee Wee League, there's no pitching at all. The players just hit the ball off a tee.

BAT AND BALL SPORTS

This has significantly reduced the number of cases of serious or permanent damage occurring to the elbow joint until Little Leaguers reach an age where the elbow muscle can effectively support the elbow joint. Recommendations have been made to further limit the amount of throwing allowed and to prevent curve-ball pitching and other more difficult pitches.

Unfortunately, there's no limitation on pitching at home and during practice. Parents and coaches should therefore be aware of the risks. Watching for signs and symptoms of elbow problems will greatly improve the chances of early diagnosis and treatment.

Good judgement and conservative measures are vital in preventing significant deformities and impairment of the elbow joint function.

Stress fractures

Stress fractures in the lumbar region of the spine are not uncommon in adolescence. They may even go unnoticed unless the individual puts a strain on the lower back and requires an X-ray of this region.

Fast bowlers in cricket often suffer stress fractures in the spine. We only have to look at such greats as Dennis Lillee, Rodney Hogg, Bruce Reid and Dennis Hickey to understand the stresses fast bowling places on the lumbar spine.

Stress fractures in the spine are difficult to treat because they are difficult to diagnose. The player may have a vague sort of back pain. Any unexplained back pain is always significant in a young adolescent who plays an active sport such as cricket or basketball. A stress fracture should always be suspected.

> **STOP**
> *Unexplained back pain is always significant.*

A bone scan will usually show up a stress fracture. A bone scan is like an X-ray only it involves injecting a radio-nuclear dye which is concentrated into areas of new bone growth or where bone has been laid down as with a fracture site.

Stress fractures are difficult to treat. The simple answer is that rest is possibly the best treatment of all. In the early days of the injury, you should rest and avoid stressing factors on the spine. Following that period of rest, a suitable exercise program is necessary to build up your fitness and important for promoting a full recovery.

An appropriate rest time would vary greatly, but for a fast bowler this could well be a whole season.

BAT AND BALL SPORTS

Don't forget the warm-up

All these sports involve a lot of running, twisting and turning. Apart from the injuries already discussed, players are liable to sustain ankle sprains, injuries to the knee joint and the commonly seen strains of the calf, hamstring and quadriceps muscles in the legs and other lower extremities.

It's therefore important for players to warm up adequately before entering the sporting arena.

The warm-up should include a stretching program specifically for the muscle groups in the legs and also the muscle groups around the shoulders, elbows and wrist joints. This significantly helps minimise muscles strain from overstress which can destroy the enjoyment of the sport.

HELPFUL HINTS

★ Always make sure that the playing field is clear of any objects and that the boundaries of the playing field are well away from fences and other immovable objects.

★ Protective equipment should be used. For example, batting gloves, groin protectors and in girls breast protection, in field hockey, correctly fitting shinpads. If a firmer ball is being used, then a protective helmet may be necessary when batting in cricket and baseball.

★ Overall, it's important that there is appropriate and consistent application of the rules in all of these bat and ball sports. Commonsense by umpires and administrators can significantly reduce traumatic injuries such as those which occur as a result of high-pitched balls in cricket.

★ The wearing of proper footwear is important in reducing skin injuries involving the sole of the feet and around the toes. Also, high-cut boots in cricket, particularly for bowlers, greatly reduces the risk of ankle sprains.

★ Always err on the side of caution if concerned about any injury. Suspect a fracture if there's any deformity or significant pain or swelling, even after the application of ice. Seek medical advice as soon as possible.

★ Overuse injuries classically occur in the shoulders and elbows of baseballers and softballers and in the mid to lower back in cricket. Preventive measures should include using Sorbathane™ in shoes and restricting a young bowler to no more than 6 to 10 overs and 10 to 14 overs in young adolescents.

Water Sports: Swimming, Surfing, Water-skiing and Sailing

6

Swimming has one big advantage over other sports. Water buoyancy reduces the gravity by 60 to 70 per cent, so swimmers don't stress their lower back and other weight-bearing joints as do runners and jumpers.

Many of the problems young swimmers encounter are caused by a combination of endurance and speed and discrepancies between a swimmer's muscle development and the performance expectations of coach and parents. By the time hard training starts, they have started their growth spurt. However, because of the difference in the growth rates of different tissues, their bones grow faster and get stronger earlier than their muscles.

It takes 12 to 18 months for the strength and stretch of the muscles to catch up to the bone strength and length. This disparity puts a lot of pressure on the muscles — in swimming or any other sport.

Growth Spurts

Girls start maturing earlier than boys and have a very rapid growth spurt. Boys catch up usually around the age of 16 to 18. This means that an 11- or 12-year-old girl can be very much stronger than a boy of the same age. A girl can usually produce greater physical effort and sustain it for a longer period than a boy. There are exceptions, of course. Some boys start their growth earlier and are stronger earlier. In general, however, girls have the edge, which explains why they compete very early in swimming and gymnastics.

COMMON SWIMMING INJURIES

Muscle strain

Muscle strain affecting the upper torso into the shoulder region is the most common type of injury for swimmers along with tenosynovitis. Swimmers strain muscles around their shoulder-blades, in the shoulders and their upper arms. They

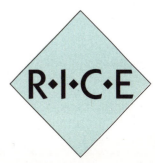

WATER SPORTS

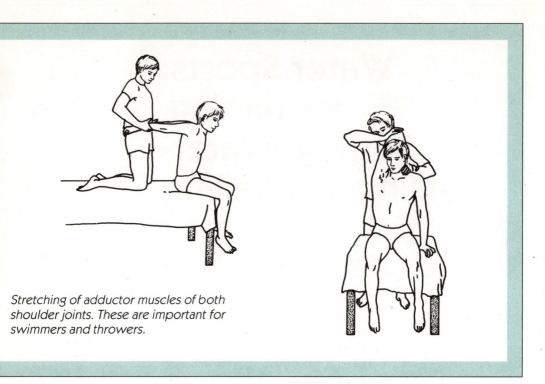

Stretching of adductor muscles of both shoulder joints. These are important for swimmers and throwers.

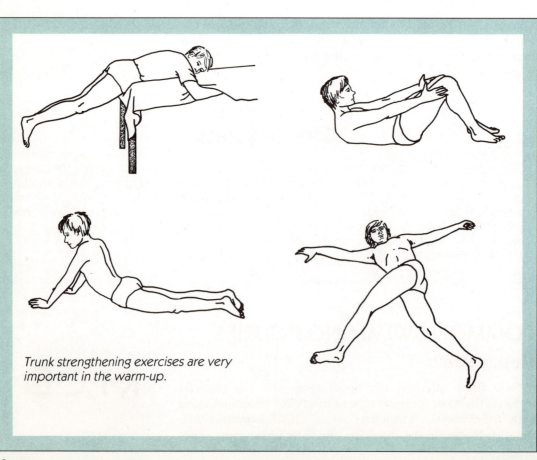

Trunk strengthening exercises are very important in the warm-up.

WATER SPORTS

also get muscle strains further down and, of course, muscle strains in their thighs and buttocks. Treatment involves applying RICE for 24 to 48 hours, followed by simple stretching manoeuvres (see page 16).

Eye infections

Children who swim regularly in pools often suffer eye irritations from chlorinated or salt-chlorinated pools. There are excellent goggles which young swimmers who do a lot of swimming can wear to avoid eye irritations. I believe goggles are now so good that they should also always be used in sea water. It's easy to get eye infections from sea water when swimming near drains emptying alongside beaches. The drains are often partly concealed, so you may not realise a potential hazard exists.

Goggles should always be worn in sea water.

It's important that eye infections are properly diagnosed. One of the best sayings is: beware of the unilateral red eye. This means a red eye on the one side and not on the other. The inflammation and redness can be due to a foreign body in the eye. Accordingly, such symptoms should always ring bells that there may be a bit of dirt, grit or even a piece of glass in the eye which could be causing the infection. No amount of antibiotics will get rid of the foreign body.

Almost invariably, if a player gets an infection in one eye it crosses to the other side. So, if they have bilateral red eyes, it's usually due to an irritation or infection. The best treatment is to keep the eyes clean and use antibiotic eye-drops.

If the eye is really irritated, you should apply an eye pad to rest the eye and every two hours apply the drops. In a day or two, it usually clears up. Medical advice should be sought about an eye infection which doesn't settle down.

Seek medical advice if an eye infection doesn't settle down.

Don't keep eye-drops for too long because they have a limited effective life. It's a good idea to keep them in the fridge. Once the infection has cleared up throw the drops away because bugs can grow in the eye-drops over a period of time.

Keep eye-drops in the fridge.

Ear infections

Ear infections are also a common problem — particularly from swimming in public pools. If children complain of earache, and if there's no external sign of ear infection, have them checked immediately by your local family GP or an ear, nose and throat specialist.

Don't keep them for too long.

Many children have problems with what is called 'glue ears', a build-up of fluid behind the ear drum (the tympanic membrane). The fluid is so thick that it doesn't drain away into

69

WATER SPORTS

the back of the throat. This is a middle-ear infection and may not be caused by swimming. The child may simply have ear problems which need treatment. Initially, try medication to drain the fluid away. In chronic cases, this won't always work. It's then appropriate to insert grommets (little tubes) into the ear drum. This increases the pressure which helps drain the gunky material down through the throat. While this solves one problem, it sometimes creates another. Once the tubes have been put in, a connection is established between the external environment and the middle ear which was previously protected by a membrane.

If the child goes swimming, fluid can flow straight through into the middle ear and cause further infection. The best way to avoid this is to get special earplugs made. The plug fits snugly into the ear. Children as young as four can learn to fit their own plugs. Some parents put Blu-Tac™ into their children's ears as well as getting them to wear a rubber swimming cap. Blu-Tac is a good, cheap method of plugging up the ear if your children are getting a lot of external ear infections from the swimming pool and you can't keep them out of a public pool because of the hot summers we have.

Sterilise earplugs in hot water every few weeks.

Children should not of course share the Blu-Tac because of the risk of cross-infections. I would recommend earplugs be sterilised in hot water every few weeks and kept in their own little containers. Children will respond well if they are taught how to use the plugs properly and realise they are not things to play with. It becomes a conditioned reflex to wear their plugs whenever they go swimming or even get into the bath.

THROW AWAY OLD MEDICINES

It's a little realised hazard with eye-drops or ear-drops that the solution in which the anti-body is held is also an ideal medium for growing bacteria.

Therefore, it's very important to keep the drops in the fridge and not to hold on to them once the expiry date is reached or the infection has cleared up. Otherwise, a few months later when your child has another eye infection and you use the old bottle, you will be putting drops now full of germs into your child's eyes or ears.

So, throw away those eye- or ear-drops as soon as your child is over the infection.

WATER SPORTS

SURFING: COMMONSENSE NOT OVERCONFIDENCE

The most important thing in prevention of surfing injuries is to surf in a safe area. No matter how great the surf looks, beware, there may be very dangerous rips, concealed reefs and unknown undertows. Wherever possible, children should always swim at a beach patrolled by lifesavers. This is ignored by numerous people of all age groups. Every year, good samaritans drown going to the rescue of swimmers in trouble at unpatrolled beaches. Lifesavers have hundreds of examples a year of near misses where they have to make rescues in treacherous stretches of surf clearly outside the marked flags. Even when swimming in a patrolled area of beach, teach children not to overlook the tried and proven buddy system. Having someone with them can make the difference of a few vital minutes until lifesavers can reach them. Cramps are just as unpredictable as dangerous undertows. No one is immune!

Also, no child should be allowed to go surfing without being a very strong swimmer. If they are out in very difficult swimming conditions, the slightest problem such as a sudden wind change could end with the child a mile off-shore before you know it. Overconfidence can be fatal. Stark and horrifying statistics confirm this every year.

When surfboard riding, ankle straps should always be used. Apart from the hassle of having to chase the board after falling off, the most important reason for wearing an ankle strap is to avoid head injuries. A surprising amount of damage can be caused by the pointed end of the board and the fin at the back when the board goes flying through the air in vigorous surf.

The strange thing is that the stray board seems to have the habit of hitting the rider more than the innocent bystander. An interesting study in California found that about 75 per cent of all head injuries to surfers were caused by their own boards! Typically, the board goes straight up and then straight down while the rider who has fallen off is being bounced around in the surf. While the people around can see the board flying and have time to get out of the way, the rider who has lost the board tends to come straight up just as the board is coming straight down!

Surf in a safe area.

Teach children to always have someone with them.

Ankle straps should always be worn.

WATER SPORTS

SURF SAFETY TIPS

★ Make sure your child is a strong swimmer and can swim unaided for at least 30 minutes.

★ Ensure that he or she wears an ankle strap. The ankle strap attached to the board and to the surfer's ankle stops the board from shooting out of control and possibly hitting either the rider or an unsuspecting swimmer.

★ Impress on your child to always surf in areas patrolled by lifesavers — no matter how tempting the surf looks elsewhere.

ENDURANCE SWIMMING

I think that all children should be able to swim constantly for at least 30 minutes. You simply don't know what can happen and I think that children should be good swimmers first before advancing to more ambitious water activities. Endurance swimming is of vital importance and should be encouraged by parents and clubs and for sailing, windsurfing and water-skiing.

WATER-SKIING AND SAILING

There are several basic rules for safe water-skiing and sailing:

★ Children must be able to swim well.
★ They must be adequately trained in how to water-ski and sail.
★ They must wear safety vests.

It really upsets me to see children water-skiing or sailing without a safety vest. I suppose it's the macho image — it's more important to look good than to wear wimpish things like a safety vest.

For sailors, there's always the danger of being hit by the boom, temporarily dazed and knocked overboard. I have first-hand experience of this. Sailing with my cousins I was once hit by the boom and almost knocked out. I woke up floating in the briny. The vest had kept my head up and saved me from certain drowning.

It is essential to have a good driver.

When water-skiing you should always be conscious of the danger of snags in dams, lakes and rivers with dead trees just under the surface. It is also essential that you have a very good driver who knows what he or she is doing. First of all, there's the risk of running into other people. Secondly, doing the wrong thing when a surprise situation suddenly confronts you.

Next, take the time to know your water-skier. How good are they and how quickly can you pull them out of the water? This particularly applies to your children's friends who may be out for the day with you.

WATER SPORTS

Always have an observer facing the water-skier at all times and not looking around like the driver. They can then efficiently tell the driver to slow down, or stop, if the water-skier is having problems. There's no other way for the water-skier to communicate to the driver that they are in real trouble.

So, it's important that you should have an experienced driver working with a good observer without a lot of distractions. Avoid having a boat full of people.

Alcohol is an absolute 'no-no'. It causes more trouble than anything else. Fuzzed co-ordination and slow reactions are an invitation for trouble.

Injuries to water-skiers are mainly shoulder soreness and back problems because of the pulling on the rope, particularly with novice skiers.

The most serious injuries occur when falling off at speed, running into a bank or hitting an underwater snag. All of these are totally avoidable. You can have pleasurable water-skiing with minimal injuries if the basic safety factors are heeded.

Always have an observer facing the water-skier.

THE DANGERS OF HYPOTHERMIA

Just a word of caution about hypothermia. I spoke earlier about the dangers of small children running too vigorously in hot weather with the risks of dehydration and hyperthermia. Children become hypothermic much more quickly than adults.

This means they can die fairly rapidly, depending on the clothes they are wearing, how cold the water is, the wind chill factor, how good a swimmer they are and how well they can support themselves if they are not using a good lifejacket or no life jacket at all.

The factor which works in children's favour is that their cardiovascular system can sustain much greater changes to their pulse rate and blood pressure. A good example of this was the recent case of the young child in the United States who fell into a frozen canal and was under water for between 10 and 15 minutes. He was floppy and blue and almost dead when rescuers pulled him out but his system had shut down so effectively that he was able to survive without long-term damage.

Children become hypothermic quickly but their cardiovascular system can sustain great changes.

WATER SPORTS

'Shut down' means that there are certain priorities which the body gives for its blood supply. Skin is the least of them. Then there's muscle and the intestines and other areas such as the kidneys. The body tries to give maximum protection to the vessels and the arteries to the brain and heart. They are the very last things the body shuts down. The body does the best it can to preserve the brain function because once the brain dies, everything dies. So, it's better to lose a few fingers or even limbs than to lose the brain!

Children have a greater ability to cope with this shut-down period than older people because of the state of their heart, their coronary vessels and the vessels to their brain.

HELPFUL HINTS

★ Do an adequate warm-up with slow stretching exercises.
★ Guard against eye and ear infections. Always use good goggles and earplugs.
★ Avoid overtraining and overstress both physically and psychologically especially with young swimmers doing heavy training sessions in the early morning before school.
★ Muscle strains and joint ligament injuries are common, especially involving the shoulders, upper back and torso. Treatment should involve the reduction of training, RICE and aspirin when necessary, followed by an exercise program.
★ Water-skiers, surfers and windsurfers should make sure they're good swimmers.
★ Check all equipment to make sure it's in good working order.
★ Know the waters you're skiing or surfing on and follow all local instructions and safety suggestions.

BMX Bike Riding, Skateboarding, Horse Riding, Snow-skiing and Ice Skating

7

While horse riding is very popular in Australia, because of the broad expanses of our countryside and our English background, the riding sports which are really booming are BMX racing and skateboarding.

The most common injury to children falling off BMX bikes, skateboards or horses is a fractured forearm or collar bone. Children are most vulnerable to falls when learning to ride. The single, most important piece of prevention advice is for a parent to be there to at least reduce the risk of a serious spill.

The biggest danger is head injuries. The answer is a proper, well-padded helmet approved by the Standards Association of Australia.

The other danger, even with a helmet, is a broken neck because the head is still free to respond to violent forces bending, or twisting, it back against the trunk.

There are no absolute answers here. All that can be done is minimise the risks by not taking unnecessary chances, building skills up to the level of experience appropriate to the manoeuvre being attempted and taking lessons in how to fall. Then practising this until it's second nature.

As BMX bike riding and skateboarding boom, so do injuries.

RIDING SAFE ON THE STREETS

For those who go for the pure enjoyment of bike riding on streets and not on competition tracks, the main thing is to make sure your bike is well maintained and especially that the foot and hand brakes are in good order. A loud bell is another necessity.

Several surveys in recent years, in New South Wales and Victoria, have revealed an alarmingly poor state of repair of schoolchildren's bicycles. Poor brakes, tyres, and rust-weakened frames are the common trouble spots.

RIDING, SKIING, SKATING

Take a close look at your son or daughter's bike and you could be jolted into doing something. Your apathy today could mean your child going under a truck or bus tomorrow. Accidents don't always happen to other people. Every day, there are hundreds of near misses to children on bikes on Australian roads.

Check that your child's bike is suited to them. An amazing number of children ride hand-me-down bikes which are too big for them. An unsteady child on a bicycle is often a prescription for disaster on crowded roads with today's deadline pressures crowding on truckies, bus drivers and motorists alike.

A tall orange flag is one of the best safety devices.

A flag is one of the best safety features available for young children riding 12 inch (30 cm) and 16 inch (40 cm) bikes, which are otherwise hard to see in streets lined with parked cars. A tall orange safety flag gives excellent high profile for a child cyclist making them immediately stand out above parked cars. The cost of around $7.50 for a flag is a cheap investment in avoiding a child being knocked off their bike when, sooner or later, they do the wrong thing.

No matter how much you train your children on a bike, situations will still arise where a combination of factors means they will have a spill. If you have taken all the proper safety precautions, then serious injury risks are minimised. It's a big help if they practise falling off their bike on to grass. BMX track coaches are excellent at falling techniques to minimise the risk of a broken arm or collarbone.

STOP
A proper SAA-approved helmet should always be worn.

The Victorian and NSW governments are to be congratulated on their campaign to get children and adults to wear helmets. The important thing about helmets is that they should have the SAA trademark that is, that they have been stringently tested by the Standards Association of Australia. This standard is frequently reviewed to see what further improvements are needed.

One of the authors of this book, Peter Fitzgerald, ran a campaign of articles from March 1980 over four years in the *Melbourne Herald* with Professor Frank McDermott of the Road Trauma Committee of the Royal Australasian College of Surgeons, the Bicycle Institute of Victoria, school teachers and bereaved parents to popularise the use of helmets for child cyclists. The Victorian government subsequently introduced a subsidy scheme to make an SAA-approved helmet an attractive alternative Christmas present to an electronic game.

RIDING, SKIING, SKATING

The then Victorian transport minister, Mr Steve Crabb, deserves credit for that breakthrough which to date has put SAA-approved helmets on the heads of more than 100 000 schoolchildren. New South Wales deserves credit for taking up the idea and also making the use of helmets widespread. The College of Surgeons estimates that this measure has collectively saved many hundreds of Australian children from either serious brain damage or death.

Other states have since shown commendable initiatives to spread the use of helmets. Apart from the human tragedy of a maimed child, the community cost of medical treatment for a seriously brain-damaged child is put at $100 000 over five years. The bicycle helmet story shows what governments and concerned doctors and parents can do to create a safer environment for children.

Improvements, of course, still need to be made. For example, try to get a helmet which is one complete shell, rather than one with the two halves fused together.

Making sure a child can be seen should be a high priority. For night riding don't forget to have a good light and reflectors on your child's bike. Again, it's paying attention to simple rules to avoid the risk of serious injury. Reflective tape is excellent for sewing onto the favourite jacket or jumper a child likes wearing at night. They should then be encouraged to carry this in their school bag, particularly in the winter months when even late afternoons mean poor visibility.

Make sure a child can be seen at all times.

It's just like seat belts. The more it becomes routine, the easier it becomes to do and the less conscious children become about doing it. Thanks to the campaigns by the Road Trauma Committee of the Royal Australasian College of Surgeons, Australians should be proud of having the highest record of seat belt-wearing in the world! It amazes people wherever we go that the first thing we do in getting into a car is to put the seat belt on. No matter if it's Yugoslavia, Britain, France or particularly the United States.

When I lived in the United States while training in specialised sports medicine operations, my medical colleagues were even more amazed to see how our children would look for a seat belt when they got into a car and put them on before the car moved off. They were really surprised about how conditioned we had become about seat belts.

RIDING, SKIING, SKATING

The most convincing argument about question of infringement of civil liberty is the tremendous improvement in the morbidity of our road accident figures. I still get angry when I see parents driving with seat belts on but allowing their children to jump around in the back seat or lying unrestrained in the back of a station wagon! Those children will become projectiles as soon as the driver has to brake hard in an emergency. The children will simply keep travelling at that speed. Unlike the car de-accelerating say from 100 kilometres per hour, the unrestrained children in the back won't! That's the speed at which they hit the windscreen and have their faces cut to ribbons.

I have seen cases of children who have gone through the windscreen and come into a hospital casualty department. The parents are not injured but the child is dead. It's hard to find words to summarise such an easily preventable tragedy.

The two key points here are that many, many more children are killed or seriously injured while riding in cars than while riding on BMX bikes, skateboards or horses. Secondly, the lesson of how putting on a seat belt has been automatically accepted as the thing to do when a child gets into a car has a tremendous significance in getting children to automatically wear a well-fitting, SAA-approved helmet in all riding sports be it BMXing (or ordinary bike riding), skateboard riding or horse riding.

TEACHING CHILDREN TO RIDE

Parents should be involved in the learning phase.

The best accident prevention device isn't on sale in the shops. It's you! Parents should be involved in the learning phase. Make the time. Being there can make all the difference between a cut or grazed elbow or a broken arm. It won't take long for the child to get enough confidence to do their own thing. Your involvement is vital in the vulnerable learning phase.

Keep children off busy streets.

Every year, the police accident statistics tell a grim story of the number of children with a new bike knocked down in January and February. So, stay off busy streets in the learning phase and stick to your backyard, driveway, a park with a bicycle track or the wide open expanses of an empty supermarket carpark on Sunday. In fact, anywhere that's flat and where they can have a spill without a sudden crisis of a car zooming around the corner.

Far too many parents are still training their children on the street. Every year, there are tragedies with cars zipping around a corner with a child suddenly in front of them.

RIDING, SKIING, SKATING

Encourage them with training wheels and then raise the training wheels slowly to allow them to develop more confidence.

It's vital that they get your help and encouragement in that initial learning phrase where they are particularly vulnerable to having a bad fall which will not only shake their confidence but often leads to a bad fracture when they instinctively put out a hand to cushion the fall.

Always beware the first two weeks back at school. The number of children killed or seriously injured leaps between Christmas Day and the end of February. A multitude of children are still unsteady on the bicycles they got for Christmas and now want to ride to and from school. There are hundreds of near misses in February with new school uniforms, strange shoes and new bikes. Combine this with a motorist running late for work and you have a prescription for disaster.

One of my bugbears with our society at present is the lack of parent involvement. I have plenty of shortcomings because of the time I spend away from my children due to the demands of the medical practice, but at weekends it really pays tremendous dividends to get involved with your children. Even when you are doing the garden, it's a great idea to get one of your young children, who is learning to ride a bicycle, to come out and ride up and down as you're doing the garden.

RIDING IN BMX CLUBS

Riding in BMX clubs is highly recommended. They're big on commonsense safety. Learning proper safety habits early on maximises injury-free enjoyment of the sport. Clubs are closely supervised with well-padded handle bars being a must for a rider to be allowed out on the track.

Another big plus is that the tracks don't have traffic hazards. Children are riding in an environment which is safe compared to roads full of unpredictable motorists involved in 'dodgem car' driving, negotiating trucks, road works and other hazards.

Children should progressively develop their skills on BMX tracks riding over jumps and moguls (little hills) and being taught how to land correctly. Such education in defensive riding is the best way to avoid injuries.

If there's no BMX track, then try to form a parents' group to approach the local council to get one. If all else fails, there's always the local park. It's better than your son or daughter learning on the road where the tuition fees could be high.

An experienced rider is necessary to teach the novice how to expertly twist and turn and achieve tremendous aerial dexterity. They have to be shown to pick up the know-how in a low-risk situation.

Then it's practice, practice, practice to perfect manoeuvres and stunts. What is a piece of cake on a proper BMX track can be inviting disaster for a BMX daredevil on a suburban street. Streets are not playgrounds. Get kids into safe areas. Don't be complacent. Know where your kids are playing and always know who they're playing with.

RIDING, SKIING, SKATING

PROTECTIVE EQUIPMENT

Protective equipment should be the cornerstone of BMX and skateboarding. That means a helmet and knee and elbow protectors for both BMX riders and skateboarders and, for BMX riders, a proper visor or goggles in races where there's a lot of dirt and mud, and wearing a good scarf like the pro-motorcyclists.

Good padding around the handlebars is important protection.

With BMX bikes it is important to get good padding around the handlebars to protect the child's teeth and groin. Skeletal injuries and groin injuries are common as the popularity of BMXing spreads. Girls are not immune from injury. Sports' medicine doctors are increasingly seeing bruising, and bleeding to the vulva (the external area around the vagina) with so many girls now engaging in BMX riding, and even just riding their brother's BMX bike, and hitting themselves between the legs with the crossbar.

Proper limb protection is particularly important for skateboard riders because they are so prone to falling off when trying new jumps on ramps. A lot of the ramps are concrete and a heavy fall on concrete is very different to falling onto a wooden surface. In skateboard riding, riders tend to land very heavily on their elbows and knees. This tends to mean bad bruising and possibly even damage to the elbow joint, the knee joint and the patella femoral joint.

For skateboarders proper limb protection is especially important.

The latter can get bruised and the cartilage of the lining on the joint can get badly damaged. Such injuries can happen in a second and can take months or years to get over. Skateboard riders should realise the tremendous stresses they are putting on their lower body, particularly below the knees, compared with their upper body which is balanced and not stretched as much.

Ankle sprains and irritations feature prominently on the casualty list for skateboard riders. They're particularly prone to Achilles problems because of the frequency of leaning over and stretching their Achilles tendon and its supporting muscles up and down.

Serious riders should always warm-up before competition.

Skateboard riders' thighs and hamstrings come a close second in vulnerability and so should be included in the warm-up. This is a basic preventive measure which cannot be over-stressed.

Any skateboard rider serious about the sport should always first do a warm-up stretch lasting 10 to 15 minutes before a competition, particularly of their calves, the Achilles and the muscles around their ankles. Doing round circles with the feet is highly recommended as well as toe and heel raises.

RIDING, SKIING, SKATING

This warm-up advice applies particularly to skateboarding but also to BMX devotees. So does wearing a proper helmet.

HEAD INJURIES

You wouldn't whack a computer on a piece of concrete, so remember your brain is vastly more delicate. Treat it with the respect it deserves. A proper SAA-approved helmet should always be worn by skateboarders. While not as good as a modern helmet, even an old-fashioned soft bicycle racing helmet is better than nothing.

With a head injury, we always talk about 'contra coup' injuries. This means that sometimes you can be hit on the back of the head but the front of the brain has been damaged or vice versa. You have to remember that the brain is suspended in fluid inside the skull. It floats. Not a lot, but there's a little bit of give in there.

If you get hit from behind, the brain is sometimes pushed forward and hits the hard part at the front. It's easy to be misled about the neurological signs of the head injury. A person may be hit at the front and is showing signs of bruising of the brain at the back and there can be bizarre signs when you're trying to work it out.

The signs of a head injury are the same in any sport. If your child has fallen off their skateboard or their BMX bike and has hit their head, ask them if they lost consciousness or remember blacking out even for a moment? Always check what part of their head they hit. This information may be invaluable later. Ask them if they have a headache, if they feel sick or if they have vomited. If you're unsure or not happy with the situation, always err on the side of being conservative and take them to the local hospital to be checked.

Take a child to the hospital if you are unsure about the injury.

Internal bleeding

A head injury may just be bruising of the brain. If it is very minor bruising the result will only be a headache. There may be some other signs but without long-term problems.

The really serious consequences are when there's bleeding into the area where the brain is situated. Remember that the brain is sitting in a solid box. So any increase of fluid into there, or any other thing which occupies space, is going to cause pressure, for example, a tumour or from bleeding.

There are two types of bleeding. Firstly, bleeding from an artery and secondly bleeding from a vein. If it's arterial bleeding, the deterioration of their brain function will be very rapid because pressure is building up from the heavy bleeding into

RIDING, SKIING, SKATING

the brain area. A person may collapse, feel nauseous, start vomiting, and show pressure on their nerves such the pupil of an eye dilating. The affected eye is usually on the opposite side of the brain to where the blood is collecting. The pupil may start getting bigger and bigger compared to the other side. Any of these signs and the child should be taken straight to hospital. I would even bypass the local doctor. He or she will only refer them to hospital immediately. Such injuries need to be treated rapidly to avoid severe long-term consequences.

Specialised tests such as X-rays and scans have to be taken immediately. Initial tests may show they have a subarachnoid haemorrhage. In simple lay terms, this means serious arterial bleeding due to the bursting of an artery or a vessel. This doesn't necessarily mean there will be bleeding from an ear or ears. Bleeding from the ear or the nose is usually only caused by a fracture at the base of the skull. Bleeding in the brain may not produce any obvious physical signs. It may just mean that it's the way the brain has been affected by that one injury, that one trauma within the skull, and an artery is bleeding.

Someone injured like this may feel fine immediately after the blow. They get up but then they can go off suddenly. When this happens, the deterioration is very rapid, within minutes. They may collapse, they may have breathing difficulties and they may need mouth-to-mouth resuscitation because of respiratory difficulties. That part of the brain which tells the lungs to work is malfunctioning. Remember the initial warning signs are dilating pupils, a very severe headache, double vision, or even collapse. If you are concerned about any of these things, the best advice is to take them straight to a medical centre. If they have collapsed, there's nothing you can really do except put all sirens on and get the patient to the nearest hospital as quickly as possible, that is, a major hospital with comprehensive facilities such as the Royal Children's Hospital in Melbourne.

> **STOP**
> *If a child has collapsed get him to a hospital quickly.*

If they're having breathing difficulties, you should apply mouth-to-mouth resuscitation. Fortunately, the respiratory centre isn't usually badly affected. This is the scenario of the fast deterioration. The most obvious one where clearly something is seriously wrong.

The other more subtle scenario is the delayed deterioration. Typically, the child comes home and says: 'I've bumped my head today, Mum'. You do a quick examination and can't see anything outwardly wrong. After a while, the headache subsides and the child says they feel alright. You relax and soon forget about it. The pressure on the brain may be building up very slowly and the deterioration is much more subtle. Then,

RIDING, SKIING, SKATING

somewhere about a week to two weeks later, your child starts to deteriorate without warning.

He or she may collapse showing the signs of an acute bleed, even though it can be up to two weeks after the injury. The culprit is almost certainly a venous leak. This simply means a vein has been damaged.

So, remember, TWO WEEKS. In the back of your mind, file away the importance of that time span. Be on the alert for any trouble your child has after a knock to the head. Typically, this could be trouble concentrating at school or amnesia. Get them to a doctor immediately. There are subtle signs indicating a venous bleed which you can look for before the child collapses and goes into that dangerous phase. Typical symptoms include some changes in the pupil and some changes in perception of light. This is because there are some nerves which deteriorate very quickly, particularly those to the eyes. The sixth cranial nerve is a nerve to the muscles of the eye which produces movement of the eyeball. It's one of the first nerves to be affected if you have some generalised pressure building up in the brain. Essentially, however, I'm saying that it's wise to play safe.

Be alert about any trouble a child has for two weeks after the injury.

If the child has had a head injury and if, over the next few days, they still feel a bit off or queasy, then get them medically examined.

The doctor will typically say, 'Because there's been a very significant blow to the head, I would like to see him again in the next few days.' This is not the doctor wanting to get another consultation fee. Rather, he wants to check for signs of what we call a subdural haemorrhage.

This advice is for coaches as well as parents. Always err on the side of getting the child checked. Someone might wonder — why are they being kept for four hours in casualty with a head injury? The answer is that they are under observation for a subarachrial haemorrhage. This will usually show up within about four hours.

Concussion

One of my pet hates in this society is the 'concussion scenario'. This is where I believe the Press has a lot to answer for along with top football administration. I will put my head right on the block and state categorically that Australians take head injuries far too lightly. This attitude is at the elite level of players, administrators and the press which moulds sporting heroes. Sports' medicine practitioners are often dismayed about how this short-sighted, complacent attitude filters right down to the junior level.

RIDING, SKIING, SKATING

The attitude is that if it's good enough for such and such a star player, then it's good enough for my little Johnnie. It's a follow on from the public reaction to a brat tennis player abusing the umpire and the idea is then popularised for a lot of kids and their parents.

Concussion is a closed head injury. (A closed injury is one where there's no cut and possibly no fracture.) Concussion is not usually a subarachrial nor a subdural injury. They are the big problems. But you still have bruising and damage to some part of the brain tissue. It may only be minor.

My policy with any football team I was the doctor for was that anyone had a serious head injury who had at least one of the following:

★ sustained a concussion significant enough either to be taken from the ground or at the end of the game had difficulty walking off;
★ was feeling sick and sometimes vomited;
★ had a headache; and/or
★ had suffered a transient loss of consciousness.

Anyone with a possible head injury should not play for two weeks.

Sometimes, the players used to try pulling the wool over my eyes because they knew my rule about anyone with a possible head injury not being allowed to play for two weeks. I am emphatic about this rule applying to kids. They should not return to BMX, skateboard riding, horse riding or placed in a position of risk because they are susceptible to even further damage if they have another fall or another knock on the head.

This may sound tough, but many neurosurgeons would say this advice still doesn't go far enough. It's been shown that, even if there's been only a very minor contusion to the brain, eye-hand co-ordination and other aspects of neurological function are still down sometimes 6 to 12 months later. You are therefore at risk not only of a further head injury but another injury if you return to a sport requiring a high level of eye-hand co-ordination, particularly a contact sport.

How many times have you read in the sports pages of a newspaper that a player with severe concussion is bravely going to play next week! This is incredibly reckless behaviour. This is the coach and the administration dictating to the medical profession, trying to get their money's worth out of a player. Such a trivialisation of head injuries is playing Russian roulette. Sooner or later, the live round must come up in the firing chamber.

RIDING, SKIING, SKATING

Sadly, Australia is not yet a truly professional football country because we still do such stupid things. Take the example of the United States where a pro-footballer or baseball player can each be worth $20 million. When I was studying specialised sports' medicine in the United States, and was with pro football and baseball teams in the major leagues, it was brought home to me again and again that the players were too valuable to put at risk. The firm rule was that any player knocked unconscious didn't play for at least two weeks and usually three weeks. If they had a second serious head injury in the same year, then they didn't play for the rest of the year. Three serious head injuries in the same year, such as being knocked unconscious or bad concussion, and they usually never play football again.

The head injury message is just as important for parents as football coaches and administrators. Never, never be blase about your son or daughter getting a blow to the head — whatever sport they are playing, or simply if they fall off their bike in the driveway or backyard.

Never be blase about a blow to the head.

Always look for any abnormal behaviour weeks after the accident and if in any doubt whatsoever, seek medical advice. A medical practitioner knows the subtle signs to look for. If this book achieves nothing else, I will be delighted if I have got across this head injury message loud and clear.

HORSE RIDING

Let's look quickly at girl horse riders who don't like wearing helmets. There's a simple way to avoid arguments. Don't give them any choice in the matter. 'No helmet, no riding!' End of conversation.

I prefer helmets without airholes. The minor discomfort of a helmet without airholes is better than the hazard of low hanging branches snagging one of the airholes and the rider being jerked off and ending up with a broken arm or broken leg or, at the worst, spinal damage.

In the final analysis, it comes back to authority and the individual. Parents and riding instructors have to be firm to be kind. A brain-damaged child on a respirator isn't a pretty sight. I have personally seen so many parents with guilt feelings about letting their child ride without a helmet that it's not easily forgotten. Marriages often break up with parents blaming one another. How do you put dimensions on such tragedy hitting a family? Wearing a helmet is just such very cheap protection. It should be nothing less than a firm condition of them mounting their horse.

RIDING, SKIING, SKATING

Fractures to the upper and lower limbs can occur in horse riding. Basically, the rider is falling from a height, usually on uneven ground and there are a lot of problems. The injuries to horse riders are similar to what we have talked about with BMX and skateboard riders.

Horse riders would do well to wear elbow and knee pads.

Horse riders would also do well to wear elbow and knee pads. Elbow pads can even be worn under a shirt. These are the simple ways of avoiding injuries. The hard truth is that a fall off any horse means considerable risk of sustaining an injury. Such injuries are usually bad bruises, contusions and fractures — particularly to the upper extremity. The most serious are head injuries.

This whole chapter is based around injury prevention, and horse riding is no exception: proper head gear, riding horses the child knows he or she is capable of riding and, if riding in a new area, first walking around it to check out whether the rider can handle the obstacles.

This is nothing less than the professionals do. The equestrians carefully check out the course. The statistical equation is that the younger a rider is and the less experienced, the better the candidate for a serious injury.

Riders have to learn to play the numbers game in reverse by minimising the risk situations, leaving only the purely accidental situations which no amount of thorough planning can foresee. The motto for every horse rider should be to expect the unexpected and to keep their mind on the job. The professionals make sure that they know the course blind so that if the horse suddenly shies at a jump and turns away to the left they don't crash into a tree around a blind bend. One reason amateurs so often get into trouble is that they haven't carefully surveyed the course and worked out a gameplan for extricating themselves from trouble at difficult sections. Practically anything can spook a horse with unpredictable consequences.

Another reason for a fairly inexperienced rider coming to grief is that they are on a strange horse which proves a little too high spirited.

RIDING, SKIING, SKATING

BOXING, HEAD INJURIES AND HELMETS

Without doubt head injuries are the number one danger in all riding sports. Boxing is a perfect example of why you should protect your head from hard blows in any sport. Boxing is a sport where the brain is subjected to sharp blows. Look at the numerous brain-damaged boxers! The human brain was simply not intended to take a series of severe shocks. That's what a hard impact is in a fall from a BMX bike, skateboard, or a horse — and that's what boxing is, no more and no less. Every time your boy gets punched in the head, his brain will just bounce in the solid bone box which is the skull.

That's why padded helmets are so important in a spill from a BMX bike, skateboard or a horse compared to a helmet with minimal padding. A well-padded helmet makes all the difference in greatly reducing brain damage.

Remember that the more the brain spins or bounces around on the spinal cord, the more chance there is of tearing arteries, rupturing veins and causing bleeding.

For these very good reasons, many doctors believe boxing is a definite 'no-no'. But, as with any controversy, there's a counterargument. In the final analysis, the simple advice is: think very carefully before you let your son or daughter take it up.

A final word of advice: don't overlook the fact that once a child has had a heavy spill, the material lining of their helmet may no longer have adequate shock-absorbing qualities.

Crash helmets should be replaced after any major impact. This precautionary move is essential even if they don't appear damaged! Taking unnecessary risks to save money can be a very expensive proposition if you're landed with a sports' injury that will sideline you for months — or maybe permanently.

This is also why a helmet is one piece of gear you should never buy secondhand. It's virtually impossible to tell whether its previous owner has been involved in a mishap. Remember, helmets have practical limitations.

In the United States where football tackling was practised with a helmet against a crush bag, mishaps were found to be unexpectedly prevalent. Often the crush bags were spring-loaded and thus accelerated against the oncoming tackle at considerable momentum. Any mistiming of the tackle meant that the neck could very easily be hyperextended or even flexed with dangerous consequences — despite the intact helmet.

STOP
Replace crash helmets after any major impact.

SNOW-SKIING

Having a high level of fitness is the biggest single factor identified by numerous studies on how to reduce the high level of injuries among novice skiers. A close second is having the right equipment, followed by going out with at least two other skiers and not taking foolhardy chances.

Be particularly careful first thing in the morning — you should be warmed-up.

Be particularly careful first thing in the morning. Are you and your children warmed up? Do you know where you're going? Are you all wearing adequate clothes? Have you checked the weather forecast? Have you let someone in the ski lodge know where you're going? Be aware of trees and check the position of pylons. It pays to carefully check the map provided before you go out. If you don't have one supplied, then ask for one.

Next, are all bindings correct? Have you checked that all the equipment is working before you go out? Don't forget ski goggles. The glare of the snow can be very treacherous. All these things are very important in preventing injuries.

Follow all directions on the mountain. If it says avalanche area, stay well clear and don't take unnecessary risks. You should always ski with a party unless you're a very experienced skier. In most situations, you should be on the mountain with people who know that you're there and know where you're going.

With more experienced skiers, injuries tend to occur either just before lunch or the last run of the day when they're tired. It's a case of the old saying that if you're up on the mountain and you're tired and you decide to have just one more run — DON'T!

Foot and ankle problems are likely with ill-fitting boots, particularly with hired equipment. Fortunately, the standard of hired equipment has dramatically improved.

The knee joint is most vulnerable because of all the twisting, turning and pivoting.

Because boots are above the ankle, they protect the ankle and subtalar joint. So, it's the knee joint which is most vulnerable because it can be severely stressed with all the twisting, turning and pivoting, particularly with novice skiers when they get their skis all twisted up and go rolling over down the slope. That's when a knee injury is most likely.

The other common injury to novice skiers is the spiral fracture of the tibia. When their skis get caught in the snow, they pivot and rotate when the bindings don't release. They are then twisting against an immovable force. Snap! They spirally fracture their tibia.

RIDING, SKIING, SKATING

Another serious risk is patella tendonitis because of the frequent bending. The forces applied to the anterior aspect of the knee joint can cause inflammation to the patella tendon.

While lower extremity injuries are more prevalent in skiers, you can also get injuries in the upper extremities. For example, 'ski stock thumb' — a painful ruptured ulna collateral ligament, which supports the joint at the base of the thumb. This can easily happen when the stock in your hand gets caught in the snow and you go forward.

Finally, a 'pro-tip' for beginners is to always tie your ski jacket around you if the weather is hot. Apart from a sudden weather change, you may get caught in a snow drift and you might be exposed overnight.

ICE SKATING

Ice skating always becomes high profile in the media when the winter Olympics are on. Children want to do it because of its grace and beauty.

Injury prevention starts with a good stretching program and keeping up a good general level of fitness with exercise. Flexibility has to be very good for a combination of endurance, speed and strength.

The most basic mistake is choosing poorly fitting boots which can cause blisters and other foot problems. Also, rolling over can cause some ankle injuries, even though they are high-cut boots.

The most basic mistake is choosing poorly fitting boots.

You should make sure that children and other novices are well supervised by a responsible adult.

Novice ice skaters should stay in the designated area so they can find their feet and balance before venturing out in the general area.

Knee and ankle pads are not usually worn but this is worth considering with the novice skater. Because of the gliding movements falling on the elbows and the knees doesn't cause as many problems as does skateboarding and BMX riding. Novice ice skaters tend to land more on their hips or bottom. They can get contusions and bruises but these are usually minimal and the standard treatment of ice gives quick relief.

RIDING, SKIING, SKATING

For the inexperienced a lesson is a good idea or at least going with someone who knows what to do. If they're falling over a lot, then make sure they are in an area that's safe, where there's not a lot of fast skating going on so, they don't get run into and get a serious injury, or get a serious laceration or even lose a finger when they fall with instinctively out-stretched hands.

With more experienced skaters, it's not uncommon to see injuries similar to skateboarding and BMXing where they are doing a lot of difficult twists and landings with heavy bruising to the elbows, knees and hips. Twisting injuries and muscle sprains are not uncommon because skaters are putting a lot of stress on their lower extremities with all the twisting and turning. They are not unlike injuries in many of the other sports and the treatment is the same.

HELPFUL HINTS

★ Know the track or course.
★ Know how to land correctly from a fall.
★ Wear correctly fitting helmets and other appropriate protective equipment such as elbow and knee protectors.
★ Never take head injuries lightly. Always seek medical advice if unsure. Don't let a child return to sport for two to three weeks if they have been knocked out or have had headaches or felt nauseated after the head injury.
★ With skiing, check the weather forecast, that the boots and other equipment are suitable for the age group, have suitable clothing in case the weather changes, let someone know which area you are going to and what time you expect to be back — and always ski in groups for safety so that someone will always be on hand to help in the event of a mishap.

Racquet Sports: Tennis, Squash and Badminton

8

The most important preventive measure in racquet sports is the use of proper footwear. Since the boom of running sports, racquet sports have been largely neglected in this area. It's only been in the last five years that the sporting companies have developed really excellent sports shoes.

Shoes are very important because racquet sports involve twisting and turning in a confined area and ankle injuries are common. Girls, particularly, have a high injury rate in all racquet sports because they play such a lot of tennis, usually wearing inadequate shoes. There was an epidemic in 1982 of chronic ankle instability in young girl tennis players. Sports' physicians found they were wearing very sloppy, loose-fitting or inadequate shoes.

Shoes are important.

It really wasn't until netball took off in Australia that people became more conscious of wearing the right type of shoes to reduce the chance of injury. Shoes then became more fashionable and thus more appealing to them to wear the right sort of shoes. Reebok and other brands became more colourful and thus more appealing to wear. This particularly applies to aerobics. But young adolescents rather than young children have got into this in a big way.

ANKLE INJURIES

Children recover quickly from an injury unlike adults and may not even have to go to see a doctor. Often, children do not even tell their parents that they have twisted their ankle. Their tissues are young, they're flexible and they're fit and although they have ankle pain with some swelling they can return to activities very quickly. If they become a little concerned, they might report this to their mother or father and then it settles down with some ice treatment and a few days' rest. But, in many cases, they don't do the proper rehabilitation.

The most serious omission, which condemns most of them to reinjury, is that they don't do an exercise program to strengthen the injured area. Furthermore, if they return too

You should always have an exercise program to strengthen an injured area.

RACQUET SPORTS

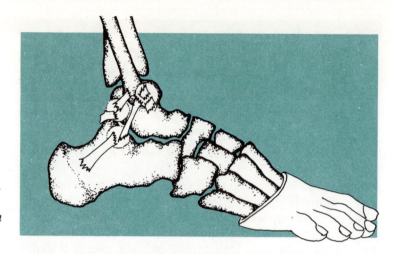

Bones and lateral (outer) ligaments of the ankle joint. The outer ligaments are the most commonly damaged in an ankle sprain.

quickly, they might just get little recurrent sprains of the lateral ligaments of the ankle and the subtalar joint, the joint just below the ankle joint. This often proves to be the straw on the camel's back and the muscles get continually weaker to the point of failure.

About the most common ankle sprain which I have referred to in other chapters is the inversion injury of the foot. The foot turns in and there is damage to the outer, or the lateral, ligament. During an examination of this injury you typically find the ligaments are a little bit lax. Possibly the most important finding is that the muscles are significantly weaker compared with the other side when you do a subjective resistance test of the muscle supporting the joint.

Testing for the strength of muscles is now much easier with specialised machines. The first was a Cybex and now there are several other excellent ones on the market which can accurately evaluate the strength of a muscle. These machines are able to test the muscles either isotonically or isometrically, and then exercise them isokinetically. The isokinetic aspect of a muscle is its strength measured against an accommodating force.

Isometric muscle strength is when you are testing the strength of a muscle against an immovable force. For example, when you are applying force through a muscle in leaning against a wall.

Isotonic muscle strength is the strength of a muscle as it's moving a weight against a variable resistance. As the weight is lifted higher against gravity, the resistance becomes greater.

The big advantage of the machines is that they give a graphic read-out and an actual value of the strength of these muscles of the knee, hip, shoulder, wrist, elbow and ankle. Thus, these machines became increasingly important in precisely assessing the level of muscle weakness.

There's also a low back machine for assessment. This has been a boon for physiotherapists and orthopaedic physicians and surgeons in improving testing and simple rehabilitation programs for the relief of chronic muscle instability. But these wonderful advances should not obscure the fact that prevention of thousands of such injuries a year is the best policy of all!

Prevention of ankle injuries comes down to two things:

★ wearing good shoes;
★ no matter how minor an ankle sprain, have it looked at and given a proper exercise program. For a child, this usually means a week for the problem to clear up.

In the early phases, a range of movement is important. Apply a resistance exercise program to avoid stiffness in the joint, particularly the ankle.

AN EASY AND EFFECTIVE ANKLE STRENGTHENING EXERCISE

A cheap and effective technique of exercising ankles is to get a new or used rubber bicycle tyre tube. Chop the valve out and then cut the tyre to make it into one long piece of rubber tube. If it's too strong for the child, cut it into just a strip of rubber and loop it at both ends similar to the old Mr Universe Exercise device. Put one loop around the foot and the other loop in your hand and work in four directions of movement: up and down at the ankle joint, and in and out of the foot by attaching it to a door or a large table.

Clearly, the tighter you pull the rubber, the harder it is. It's a very simple but very effective technique. The young athlete starts gradually and works strongly over a two- to three-week period. This is the most common and the simplest way to avoid unnecessary complications.

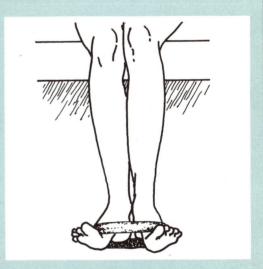

Shin muscle strengthening exercise using a segment of tyre tubing. This is an excellent exercise following ankle sprains.

The problem of chronic ankle instability shouldn't exist in children and young adolescents by following this simple rule: if a child gets an ankle sprain treat it correctly, quickly and efficiently.

Treat an ankle sprain correctly, quickly and efficiently.

RACQUET SPORTS

If you suspect that a child has a tendency to fall over, or otherwise have any problem with their ankle, then you should have them checked. An exercise program is also advised to strengthen their forehand before they start playing tennis.

WARM-UPS ARE ESSENTIAL

A warm-up is essential in all racquet sports. It's very simple to just go onto the court, start playing and doing 'a hit up'. That's not the proper warm-up needed to avoid injury. Proper exercises have to be done to adequately prepare muscles and joints.

In tennis, squash and badminton, the vital areas to work on are the tendo-Achilles, the shoulder and upper limb muscles. In particular the elbows and wrists should be flexible enough to give them a range of movement up and down. In general, get the muscles working.

Elbows and shoulders should be worked through the full range of movement. Forwards, moving from the side, extending slowly, and then stretching the quads and the hamstrings of the thigh muscles.

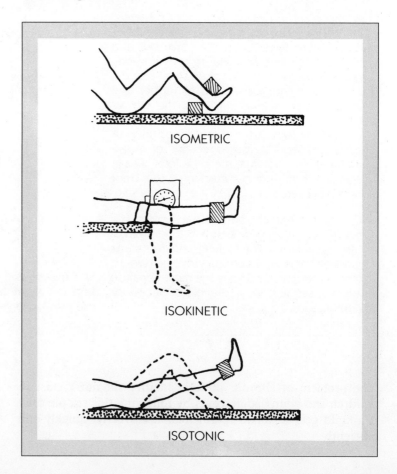

Strengthening exercises for the hamstring and quadriceps muscles. These show the three modes of exercise for muscle strengthening.

RACQUET SPORTS

COMMON INJURIES
Avulsion injuries

Racquet sports are notorious for tendo-Achilles problems — either a partial or complete rupture. Mainly adults suffer this because they're playing vigorously. Children tend to be more flexible. They get more of an irritation of their tendo-Achilles. The other important point with the younger players is that tendons, particularly near the attachment to bone, are stronger.

The consequence for children is a greater chance of an avulsion of a ligament or tendon around a joint. An avulsion is when either a ligament or a tendon, instead of rupturing when the force is applied, tends to pull off where it's attached to the bone. This is because a tendon or ligament is usually stronger than the bone in the area where the tendon is attached.

With children it's common to see such an avulsion injury in the tendo-Achilles or ligaments around the knee and elbow.

Racquet sports are notorious for tendo-Achilles problems.

Heel injuries

In young males between 11 and 14 years, it's common to see Sever's Disease with the secondary growth plate on the heel bone becoming irritated or inflamed.

Children with this condition don't always stop playing because they're so resilient. The problem just builds up. When the discomfort gets too much to put up with, they tell their parents who seek medical help. The doctor invariably finds a history of running long distances, or that they've been on a long hike or have been playing a lot of tennis, squash or netball on a hard surface.

These injuries to the heel are usually jarring injuries. Children get pain and a gradual limp. The pain is aggravated by low heels, standing on tip toes and when pressure is put on the back of heels. Usually the doctor does an X-ray and this might show some changes in the growth plate. The symptoms are usually short-lived and recurrences are common until the growth plate is finished.

Injuries to the heel are usually jarring injuries.

The treatment is to relieve the tension on the growth plate and this means using a heel pad to elevate the heel a little. Alternatively, strap the foot to hold it in a position where the heel is raised to take the pressure off their growth plate. As mentioned earlier this can be a common thing in boys 11 to 14. So, when they present with heel pain, the doctor should suspect Sever's Disease, or a tendo-Achilles inflammation.

RACQUET SPORTS

A CAUTIONARY TALE

The following cautionary story applies equally to children as well as to adult squash players. I was a young doctor on night duty in a casualty department of a large public hospital in Melbourne when two injured squash players were brought into casualty. They were good mates but had become pretty intense about their squash. One presented in casualty with a black eye and a broken nose. The other was badly bruised about the face.

I was curious about why they had such a bad fight on the squash court. As I was patching one of them up for a broken knuckle I got the blow-by-blow description of how they had hit the walls as they fought and rolled around. He said, 'I really don't know why it happened. My mate suddenly went crazy and started thumping me!'

So, I went into the next cubicle and started to treat his companion's head injuries. He was in a fair amount of pain and he started moaning and groaning. 'Why did you start it?' I asked him.

'My right leg was killing me around the calf area. That's what happened. I was playing a shot and he was behind me and he kicked or hit me with his racquet right at the back of my leg. I was in agony so I turned around and thought that, because I was beating him, he was getting narky and had decided to have a go at me.'

When I examined his leg I found that he had completely ruptured his tendo-Achilles. When that happens it can be like a pistol shot, the pain is so intense.

Anyone in this situation could be excused for thinking that their opponent had either kicked them hard in the back of the leg or whacked them with a racquet. This rather innocent on-court injury led to them both ending up in casualty. But the most serious injury of all remained the ruptured tendo-Achilles!

This misunderstanding and instant suspicion of your opponent, even in a friendly game of squash, is more common than most players realise.

A total rupture of the tendo-Achilles needs to be sutured fairly quickly. This injury can be missed by young players and sometimes even their doctors. The classic test is to lie them on their stomach with their feet hanging over the edge of the bed. A doctor only has to run his finger down to find the problem because the tendo-Achilles is such a lovely, firm tendon that the break is just so definite.

RACQUET SPORTS

Upper limb injuries

Injuries to the upper limbs are a significant problem with players of racquet sports. The major ones are shoulder injuries, especially rotator cuff irritation. The rotator cuff is the common group of tendons of muscles which produce the rotatory movements of the arm at the shoulder joint. Inflammation of one or several of these muscles, particularly in the tendons, can cause pain when the arm is being moved up or from the side and rotating it. For example, in serving in tennis.

This injury occurs mainly because of overuse when playing a lot of tennis. In tennis, players tend to hit from the elbow with the wrist firm. They use more of their elbow and shoulder. So, it's probably more common in tennis and also in badminton because badminton also involves a lot of overhead movements.

It's less common in squash because there are fewer overhead movements. Squash is a more wristy sport than tennis. Players tend to hit vigorously from the side. If they are playing good squash, then the wrists and forearms can take a surprising amount of punishment without the player realising it. In squash, therefore, inflammation of the capsule and ligaments in the wrist can occur. Again, the treatment is rest, ice and maybe taking some anti-inflammatory medication.

If a shoulder injury persists, it may be worthwhile contemplating some long-acting local anaesthetic or a cortisone injection into the bursa (the sac which is bathing the area with fluid around the common tendon group). This is a very effective way of getting an anti-inflammatory into that area.

Rotator cuff irritation is common in tennis and badminton.

Wrist injuries are common in squash.

RACQUET SPORTS

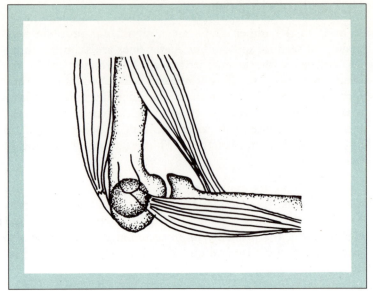

Tennis elbow is commonly a combination of inflammation to the outer aspect of the elbow joint especially involving the origin of the extensor muscles.

Cortisone injections, if used correctly, are usually very effective provided they go into a space bathing a tendon and not into a tendon or a muscle itself. Cortisone is a very effective anti-inflammatory. It works by reducing the natural tissues' inflammatory response. This in turn allows the tissues to heal and recover. So, if it's injected directly into a tendon the area becomes very weak and can eventually rupture.

It's wise to consult a sports' medicine specialist if your GP hasn't had a lot of experience with a resistant tennis elbow or rotator cuff inflammation, particularly in treating a young adolescent, and if the condition hasn't resolved itself with normal treatment methods or physiotherapy.

Tennis elbow

Tennis elbow is a significant problem with young tennis players although probably not as prevalent as it is with adults. Tennis elbow is classically the description of pain over the outer, or lateral, aspect of the elbow joint. It gained its name because it was very common in tennis players, caused by the forces generated by their backhand. Backhand movements require extension of the wrist or firmness of the extensor muscles. The lateral aspect of the elbow joint is the origin of the extensor muscles to the wrist. Thus, a traction injury can occur when applying a very strong force to this area. This can cause inflammation of the actual bone which is called lateral epicondylitis. It can also cause tenosynovitis of the muscle origin. Inflammation of a small joint between the humerus bone of the upper arm and the radius, a forearm bone, can also cause pain and restrict movements of the elbow and forearm. A proper warm-up is the biggest preventive measure against tennis elbow.

A proper warm-up is the best method of prevention.

RACQUET SPORTS

One of the most overlooked preventive measures, which is now starting to get the attention it deserves, is the type of racquet used. A child should never use a racquet with the wrong grip size. It's been found that the way a player grips the racquet has a great effect on the tension of the muscles in the forearm.

There's a similar problem on the inner aspect of the elbow known as medial epicondylitis. This is commonly known as 'golfer's elbow' because the way they hit the ball causes an inflammation of that area.

It's really not the weight of the racquet which is critical here. Rather, it's the size of the grip. The important thing is to make sure that, when you're buying a racquet, price isn't the only criterion. It's important to buy from a place where they measure the child's hand to make sure the grip size and weight is right. It's also vital that the racquet should not be of a design that's inherently heavy.

There was a rapid increase in the prevalence of tennis elbow when a larger, oversize racquet head became popular and the average tennis player rushed to get it. With certain types of racquet with an oversize head, the weight ratio from the head of the racquet down to the grip wasn't quite right. A lot of players were getting tennis elbow because of the imbalance. Always check for any warning signs of inflammation around the joint because an early presentation of tennis elbow can be treated very effectively with proper management and exercises.

A child should never use a racquet with the wrong grip size.

EXERCISES FOR TENNIS ELBOW

There are three exercises which I think are basic for minimising the effects of tennis elbow and should be used by people who have had problems. Firstly, put the forearm flat on the desk or the table and do a hand clench with your wrist. Then, bend your wrist down and back, up and down, up and down. Do at least 20 of these.

Secondly, put your elbow bent onto your head and do straightening and bending, working on your triceps muscle on the back of the upper arm.

Thirdly, I think the best exercise is one we devised at the Malvern Sports' Medicine Clinic, in Melbourne. We used to call it the 'Tennis Elbow Stretch'. It involves putting the back of your hands together, just as if you are going to do a breast stroke.

Keep the back of your wrists together and pull your hands back, keeping them straight. You can feel the tension on the muscle there as you go out. Now pull back. You hold this position until the count of 10 and then just relax. Do 20 of these.

I think such an exercise is important for anyone in the early stages of the treatment. So is the use of frictional massage, ice massage and possibly an anti-inflammatory.

You can do a combination of frictional and ice massage: by applying the ice you are doing a form of frictional massage. Also, do some friction with your fingers by simply rubbing over the area where the tendon, or the origin of the muscle, is on this bony part of your elbow.

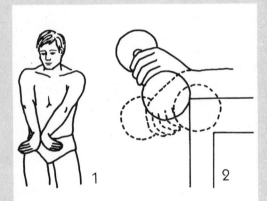

1 Tennis elbow stretching exercise for both elbows. The elbows and the hands are kept straight. The hands bend out at the wrists. Keep the back of the wrists together until pain is felt at the outer elbow region.
2 Strengthening exercise for the forearm extensor muscles using either a dumbbell or a convenient weight such as a sock filled with sand and weighing about 5 kilograms.

EYE INJURIES

Eye injuries are common in squash and badminton. Any sport where a missile is smaller than the eye socket deserves commonsense precautions. You can be hit by a tennis ball and it can really irritate your eye but the ball is bigger than the bony socket. So it can cause some damage but the small risk makes it unnecessary to wear goggles.

The really big danger is the squash ball which can move at up to 190 kilometres per hour, and has a big potential for massive eye injuries because it is smaller than the eye socket. It can therefore hit the eyeball directly without any reduction in its velocity.

RACQUET SPORTS

The eye sits in a bony box and, if you apply a rapid increase in the force within that bony box, something has to give. Either the eye will rupture, or one of the walls will rupture, and it's usually the floor. Known as a 'blow out' fracture, the eye can squeeze down through the floor of the orbit.

The result is a sunken eye as well as significant damage to the nerves of the eye, particularly the optic nerve of the eyeball. This can be permanent and may even cause blindness if the optic nerve has been severely damaged.

I see this as a potential danger across the whole age range. But, while children playing squash are not going to hit the ball as fast as an adult, it's an excellent idea to start them wearing goggles. When they go to play squash, they put on shoes, sweat band and eye goggles. Wearing them should become such second nature that they feel odd without them.

The danger is compounded by squash being in such an enclosed space that the ball can come at a player from really odd directions. It can bounce off any of the four walls as well as the floor. Thus, it's mandatory in squash that you wear proper protective goggles at all times no matter what age group.

Protective goggles are a must in squash.

In tennis, there is a much greater chance of avoiding the ball because there is usually time to take evasive action unless, of course, the ball is smashed straight at the player.

In badminton, protective eye gear is a good idea but isn't as essential. The shuttlecock certainly doesn't go as fast as a squash ball. The feathers slow it down. But, in top grade badminton, you do occasionally see the players wearing goggles because the end of the shuttlecock is smaller than the eye socket.

CONCLUSION

The key things in these sports are that they are very intense and use a surprising number of muscle groups in your lower and upper limbs.

Watch the footwear because players are doing a lot of twisting and turning. At the first sign of ankle strain, treat it effectively by supplementing the healing process with regular exercises to strengthen muscles which support the ankle and the foot.

Watch for heel irritation, involving the growth plate of the heel bone, particularly in boys. It can also occur sometimes in girls. Commonly, look at the tendo-Achilles which can become inflamed in all jumping sports and may rupture. But this tends to be more of a problem for older players in tennis, squash and badminton.

RACQUET SPORTS

Shoulder injuries are probably more prevalent in tennis and a little less in badminton and rarer in squash which tends to have injuries involving the wrist and the forearm and can include the elbow.

One other important thing in squash is that players are running and twisting and turning and bumping into walls. Concussions and injuries to the arms and the legs can occur from being hit by a racquet, or from running into a wall. Rubber walls are not yet a practicality!

The cornerstones of treatment are again ice, rest, anti-inflammatories and, if the injury is resistant, particularly with rotator cuff injuries in tennis, they may require an injection of corticosteroid (a combination of cortisone and a steroid) and local anaesthetic. It's important to understand that this is never injected into a tendon or into a muscle because it can cause rupturing. It's advisable to put it into a space such as a joint.

With all racquet sports a warm-up is essential.

With tennis elbow, the important factors are a proper warm-up using specific exercises, and carefully checking a child's racquet for weight and grip size and the size of the head.

When playing all racquet sports remember to warm up correctly, wear suitable shoes, use only well-chosen equipment and treat all injuries, no matter how slight, in the appropriate way.

HELPFUL HINTS

★ Always allow enough time for a good stretching warm-up.
★ Match the racquet to the child. Remember the:
  size of the racquet head: a normal size head for juniors, a mid-size head for adolescents and young adults and usually the veterans play with an oversize racquet.
  type of racquet: usually wood for under the age of 12, wood or aluminium for 12 to 16 and then after that into your graphites and ceramics.
  grip size to match the size of the hand.

★ With small ball sports, such as squash and racquet ball, always wear protective eye glasses.
★ Injuries commonly involve the upper extremities, the shoulder, elbow and wrist, as well as the lower leg, particularly tendo-Achilles inflammation.
★ The return to activities after injury should be graduated and involve a co-ordinated exercise program to strengthen the involved muscle groups.

Netball and Basketball

9

Basketball and netball are two big success stories of the sports scene in many countries. The National Basketball League is going from strength to strength with aggressive recruiting campaigns in schools boosting the numbers of players every year. Netball is probably the most widely played sport by women. Until recently, Australia was the world champion. For example, in Australia, an estimated 750 000 women and girls play netball.

In such fast-moving and exhilarating games, injuries are inevitable. However, the emphasis on treating sports injuries is often woeful. This particularly applies to netball. Many injuries, if not most, go untreated. A tremendous improvement is needed. There should be absolutely no compromise — all injuries, minor as well as serious ones, need prompt attention.

> **STOP**
> *All injuries need prompt attention.*

I remember a late afternoon I spent at Melbourne's Royal Park. A sports' trainer friend had asked me to go along to a mid-week match because he was concerned they didn't have any sports' medicine advice. I thought I would volunteer an hour of my time because there would only be a few teams playing. Instead, I was amazed at the hundreds of girls in action! It was one of the major regional areas that play netball every night of the week. There were numerous games going on simultaneously, playing constantly and rotating around. The vigour, zest and enthusiasm were infectious.

I set up a mini-clinic there with my sports' trainer friend. Within an hour, we had looked at eight girls who had sustained major knee injuries over the past few days. Then, in that first hour, there were six new injuries! They were the common injuries I talk about in this chapter — injuries to ankles, knees and fingers.

PREVENTION

Any large regional netball or basketball centre should have a physiotherapist or sports' trainer on hand.

In view of the sheer numbers of netballers and basketballers, it's a tremendous service to have a trained person present to provide first aid treatment and to know when to refer a more serious injury to an appropriate sports' medicine doctor, or medical specialist if it's a really tricky injury.

NETBALL AND BASKETBALL

Efforts have been made to deal with the lack of qualified personnel. There are now many good sports' trainers at level 1 and level 2 as set by the Australian Sports' Trainers Association, together with the Australian Sports' Medicine Federation. Both organisations are to be commended for their efforts to improve sports injury prevention and treatment.

Parental involvement

If your children play these sports, you, as a parent, can become involved and help improve the existing inadequate situation. As many parents as possible should learn basic first aid. Parents who attend games regularly should make sure there's a roster of people who have a first aid certificate. At every game, there should be someone available who can not only administer first aid but also recognise a more serious injury needing the attention of a doctor or hospital.

As many parents as possible should learn basic first aid.

Every parent and club official should know how to use RICE — rest, ice, compression, elevation — and also know that heat should never be applied to an injury. All heat does is promote bleeding and cause complications.

The court

Because basketball and netball are played on regular-sized courts they can be surveyed fairly quickly. It's important that the boundaries of the court are well marked and not close to fixed objects which players can run into.

Many basketball courts are squeezed into a small hall with little room between the boundary line and the wall. Consequently, players concentrating on watching the ball can run slap bang into the wall causing considerable injuries. At the very least, remove large objects such as tables and chairs.

A sweaty floor is dangerous so make sure that the court is constantly being wiped down.

Sweat is the hazard in all sports played on floors, particularly basketball. A surprising amount of sweat and moisture is generated in a game. A 'sweaty' floor can easily cause a slip resulting in a significant injury to the back or a twisted ankle or knee. So, always make sure that the court is wiped down before, during and after the game when playing on a polished floor.

Both basketball and netball can be played indoors or outdoors. When outdoors, they unfortunately tend to be played on asphalt which can be mighty rough stuff. It can be hard on the feet, particularly on a hot day. Falling can mean a graze and an infection. You must be careful to get any wound cleaned thoroughly.

NETBALL AND BASKETBALL

Protective pads

I don't think it's overly cautious to have children wearing BMX-style elbow and knee protection pads. With volleyball, the same principles apply.

You see more and more top-level basketballers wearing protective kneepads. Landing on the knee can damage the lining. The cartilage on the undersurface of the kneecap can be cracked and cause irritation and other problems. This happens in netball, basketball and in volleyball.

Landing on the knee can damage the lining.

Shoes

Netball produces a fair number of girls with significant knee injuries. Some people believe wearing high-cut shoes — that is, above the ankle joint — puts more stress on the knee joint.

I disagree because stresses on the knee joint are different from those on the ankle and cause totally different injuries. Thus, I believe protecting your ankle by strapping or with high-cut boots doesn't make the player any more vulnerable to knee injuries.

In basketball, netball and volleyball, there's a tendency to get ankle injuries with so much twisting and rolling over on the foot. Girls playing these sports should consider wearing higher cut shoes to protect their ankles. The time-honoured shoe in these sports has been a low-cut black shoe made by Dunlop. However, there are now a greater variety of shoes being worn. While most are low cut for reasons of speed, children can still get a pair of high-cut shoes to provide that all-important ankle support.

Girls should wear high-cut shoes.

Most basketballers now wear a high-cut boot to protect their ankle joints to prevent recurrent ankle injury. You only need to look at the National Basketball League in the United States and Australia to see that the majority of players wear high-cut boots. It's heartening to see this tendency filtering down into the minor leagues setting the right example for young players.

INJURIES
Knee injuries

In netball, the knees are placed under tremendous stress when the player has to catch the ball, stop quickly and perhaps pivot. It's these movements which can damage the internal structures of the knee: the meniscus (the cartilage) and the cruciate and collateral ligaments.

NETBALL AND BASKETBALL

Knee injuries are also common in basketball. The twisting, turning and sudden stopping, jumping and landing can put stress on the knee joint. The anterior aspect of the knee, the patella tendon, can become inflamed above and below the kneecap and the patella femoral joint can become irritated.

The knee is an area always to watch. (See Chapters 2 and 3 for a full discussion of the on-the-spot knee injury treatments.) Long-term treatment again means looking at the factors which predispose children to such injuries. The injured child could have what is commonly called 'jumper's knee' which is a term like 'tennis elbow'. In such a case, it's wise to get several different diagnoses of anterior knee pain.

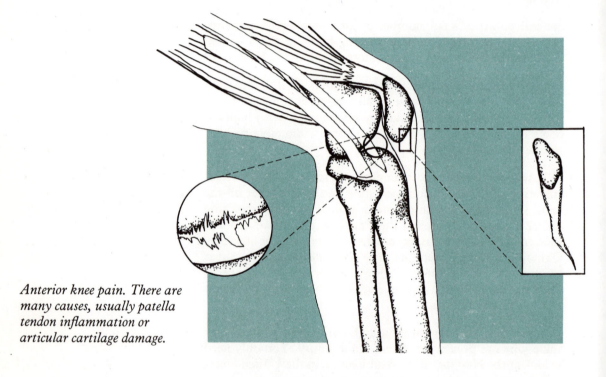

Anterior knee pain. There are many causes, usually patella tendon inflammation or articular cartilage damage.

The pain might be caused by tenosynovitis or irritation on the undersurface of the kneecap. It could be a stress fracture to the patella, or perhaps inflammation to the outer covering of the patella. It could be any of a whole range of different conditions.

Osgood-Schlatters syndrome

One of these possibilities is Osgood-Schlatters syndrome. This is inflammation and possible separation of the patella tendon from the growth plate where the tendon attaches to part of the lower leg bone. The point of attachment is a protuberance known as tuberosity. There's a secondary growth plate in the tibia at this tuberosity. Varying degrees of inflammation occur, graded 1, 2, 3 or 4 depending on how far the area of bone has been pulled off the growth plate.

In children between 11 and 14, particularly the athletically involved, this can become a serious complaint because of the rapid pulling of the tendon when they run or jump.

Treatment for the disorder used to be immobilisation by putting the limb a plaster cast for eight weeks. While this certainly settled the inflammation down, doctors found that the inflammation and consequent pain reappeared when the young athlete went back to normal activity.

The patient has to expect a period of pain and the doctor and patient just have to work together at this difficult time because it's a problem that takes a while to heal.

The treatment nowadays involves modifying the activities. The child is encouraged to participate but to limit this activity so as not to cause too much pain. After any such activity, the affected area should be given an application of ice. The child is also given exerises to strengthen the quadriceps muscles.

Initially, anti-inflammatory medication may also be needed as it's quite a painful injury and they may need a period of rest.

The aim is to build them back to enough activity to keep them happy and going, but not too much to cause irritation to the injury. Children suffering from this complaint should see the doctor every three to six months and should be re-examined after their adolescence.

This particularly applies to those who have a chance of getting into problems because the injury has involved the tendon being pulled off a fair way, often resulting in an operation to screw the piece of bone back to a better position. Fortunately, only a small minority need such care.

However, they should not contemplate a return to their sport until the growth plate has finished growing. Then, if the bone is still off, if it hasn't been attached properly, it can be screwed back in.

Screws, plates or pins should never be put across a growth plate. This effectively destroys the blood supply to that area and can cause premature closure of that growth plate.

NETBALL AND BASKETBALL

Always be wary when knee pain persists.

Other knee injuries

Serious knee injuries, such as torn cartilages, can mimic pain in the knee. Always be wary when knee pain persists. If there is any clicking in the joint or if the joint catches when walking or running, then you should be wary about a condition called 'internal derangement'. It could be a damaged meniscus, the consequence of which could be damage to the joint's cartilage.

With the advent of arthroscopy, the complaint is not difficult to investigate and simply correct in its early stages. This complaint usually involves a persistently painful knee which may affect children's school work and their efforts to do daily physical activity as well as sport.

If there's a torn cartilage in an area where the doctor believes the blood supply is still possible for healing, he might perform a meniscoplexy. This is the repair of a torn meniscus by sewing it back together. If the damage is more peripheral, towards the edge of the meniscus, the doctor might just remove the torn part, and the patient will get no further clicking or irritation of the joint.

However, if there's damage of the cartilage, a doctor may be able to pin it back into place to promote healing or, if the injury is more superficial, scrape off the damaged cartilage and smooth the area over.

A basketballer or a netballer who lands heavily and has twisted their knee often feels no pain in the very early phases, even if they have completely ruptured their knee because of the complexity and the unusual aspects of the nerve supply to the ligaments. Although they may feel a bit wonky and have to be taken off the court, they typically say, 'Oh, I've probably only just jarred my knee. I think I'm alright. It hasn't really started to swell or anything. I feel like going back on.'

This is now a very good time to make a manual examination of the knee. The injured child is not feeling a lot of pain so the muscles haven't gone tight to protect the knee. You may detect a complete damage to the anterior cruciate ligament.

Rapid swelling at the knee is caused by bleeding into the joint and is called haemarthrosis.

If the knee starts swelling rapidly, the swelling is due to bleeding into the joint. This is called a haemarthrosis and it means that something in the joint which has a blood supply, such as a ligament or a cartilage, is either fractured or torn and the blood is going into the joint. The result is a rapid collection of fluid over the next 30 minutes to 2 hours.

If the knee swells over perhaps 12 hours it's more likely to be a 'synovial effusion', that is, the lining of the joint has been irritated and this in turn causes a build up of fluid. The more information you have, the better, because you don't want to

NETBALL AND BASKETBALL

miss a major knee injury such as damage to an anterior cruciate ligament or to a collaterate ligament.

If you are not near a medical facility and the concern is that a player has twisted a knee awkwardly, never let the child back on to the field. A knee injury that causes a player to be unable to get up and walk, or return to play, must be considered a major knee injury until proven otherwise.

The guideline to follow is to observe the knee for the next few hours. If it rapidly swells, then you have a major knee injury. If it swells over the next 24 hours, you still may have a major knee problem. Use an appropriate medical centre for assessment with X-rays to check for a fracture or an avulsion of the anterior cruciate ligament.

Eventually, the child will end up with a normal knee again. But, if the anterior cruciate ligament has been ruptured, then it's important to know that as early as possible. Reconstructing a knee can be tricky and it's something to avoid if possible.

Giving the surgeon and treating physicians as much information as possible about the injury allows for different treatment alternatives. The important thing is to get a knee injury seen early, that is, in the first seven days.

If a medial or lateral collateral ligament is injured and there's undue delay in seeking medical treatment, by the time the doctor sees it the ligament may have retracted too much for the doctor to sew it back together. In the first few days, if a doctor has the option to repair it, the patient has a much better chance of a full recovery. You can go to the GP rather than a specialist for that first assessment.

HELPFUL HINTS

★ Check the court out. Make sure that the boundaries are well away from large immovable objects such as walls, posts, kiosks, tables, chairs so that they don't run into them. This also applies to other sports in relation to the boundary line.

★ A warm-up is very important. Stretch the lower limbs: the muscles, the thighs, the hamstrings, the calves. Don't forget the lower back. Athletes doing these sports are using a lot of muscle groups so it is important to be flexible, particularly with the upper body.

★ Wear the right shoes, particularly high boots in basketball and possibly also in netball. Elbow and knee protectors give adequate protection for a heavy landing, particularly in volleyball. This also applies to basketball and netball. With outdoor courts, grazes to knees and elbows are very common.

★ Be aware of the potential for injuries to the lower limbs, especially to the knee and its ligaments.

10 Strength Sports: Gymnastics and Weightlifting

GYMNASTICS

Success in gymnastics calls for not only natural ability but long and gruelling practice sessions, sometimes twice a day, six days a week. The effects of such intense training should never be overlooked if serious, nagging injuries are to be avoided.

With surprisingly little publicity, Australia is headed for major success in gymnastics. The sport is booming because of an extensive recruiting drive in schools in recent years in all states. Girls are particularly attracted to gymnastics because of its disciplined grace and elegance and its close affinity with calisthenics.

Flexibility and strength are of paramount importance in gymnastics because of the very strenuous programs involved. In particular, considerable strength is needed in the lower body and the back, and in the development of good wrists and shoulders.

Stress applied is not only during routines on the uneven bars, but floor routines, jumping and tumbling also put stress on the back and shoulders and upper limbs and extremities as well as knees and ankles.

Long-term problems can develop through overuse.

Long-term problems can develop through overuse, because gymnasts become good at a very young age. It's possible for a 13- or 14-year-old to represent their country internationally. Such high expectations impose tremendous stress on these children with the amount of training they have to do. Overuse syndrome (fully discussed in Chapter 2) should and can be prevented.

More injuries can happen in training than in competition.

It should be remembered that in sports such as weightlifting and gymnastics more injuries happen in training than in actual competition. In training, children are practising difficult routines not quite perfected and may be fighting physical and mental fatigue, so making them vulnerable to injury. Coaches and athletes must be on the alert for such warning signs that there may be an injury around the corner. They have to be careful with new routines until children build up the necessary strength.

110

STRENGTH SPORTS

The most common injuries in gymnastics

The most common injuries I would see in child gymnasts are:

★ problems in the patella femoral joint pertaining to the patella tendon around the insertion of the tibial tuberosity;
★ irritation of the growth plates at the elbow and knee; and
★ problems also with tendonitis around the elbows, and also in the shoulders (not unlike weightlifting but for different reasons).

Gymnastics is a strength sport and involves tremendous forces being applied to the body in different ways.

With girls, there's also the possibility of spinal problems. Although they have great flexibility, they can get irritation in the ligament capsules supporting the vertebral joints. This is fairly common in gymnasts but fortunately such injuries are not usually serious ones.

Joint injuries, however, can be quite disabling or cause significant deformities. As distinct from other contact sports, they are mainly due to overuse rather than from overstress. With appropriate treatment, such as resting the area and stretching exercises, they usually overcome them and quickly resume training and competition.

Most joint injuries are caused by overuse.

Age and training in gymnastics

In a sense, some children start gymnastics in a play situation at the age of three or four. Then they just build up from there. Even at this early age there's need for good coaching to ensure a sound progression of activities. It then all comes down to their capabilities physically, and to some extent emotionally, about how much training they can tolerate.

I discussed in Chapter 1 how unrealistic training expectations can affect the emotional and psychological development of young athletes. Not only is their sport affected. So is their family life, their relationship with their peers at school and their mental calm and ability to cope with problems which are part and parcel of today's stressful lifestyle. Children can also be surprisingly well tuned to any tensions in their home environment and any feelings of insecurity can have a major effect on their sporting performance.

All of these things are important and should be carefully assessed by the coach and parents if the child athlete is to progress quickly to a high level of achievement at an early age. To do this, they need tremendous dedication, iron-clad self-discipline to stick to a strenuous training program, a burning desire to succeed and they need to be prepared to cheerfully make tremendous sacrifices especially in denying themselves a proper social life.

STRENGTH SPORTS

HORMONAL MANIPULATION

Hormonal manipulation is definitely rearing its head. In Australia it is not a major problem yet but the dangers should be recognised now before it becomes prevalent.

Manipulation for suppressing hormone levels by chemical means is illegal but widespread, not so much in Australia but certainly in the Eastern European countries. If such techniques are available, some people will always be tempted to use them no matter how irresponsible it is. The long-term effects of these drugs are not yet understood, but research work has started to investigate possible side-effects.

Most sports' medicine doctors would have stories to relate from their casebooks. The best one from my experience was with a mother and daughter who came in to see me. The mother stunned me when she remarked that everything pointed towards her daughter being a champion gymnast over the next three or four years, if only her puberty could be delayed. 'The problem is to make her strong and small. I read in a magazine recently about boosting sporting performance by hormonal manipulation and I'm wondering if you can help.'

After recovering from my amazement, I tried to dissuade her. But they left clearly dissatisfied and very likely to continue their 'doctor shopping'.

While I don't believe this irresponsible attitude is prevalent in our society, I believe that it will be unless we are alert to the ever-increasing pressures for athletes to push themselves to the very limits of their physical abilities. We can expect that hormonal manipulation to boost performance will inevitably become a serious problem with people so blinded by the promise of sporting glory that they ignore the large question mark about long-term safety to their health.

STRENGTH SPORTS

> ## WARM-UP EXERCISES FOR GYMNASTS AND WEIGHTLIFTERS
>
> A warm-up program is vital for both gymnastics and weightlifting because adequate preparation of the particular muscle groups is necessary as both sports involve putting muscles under so much stress.
>
> With weightlifters, I advise them to work on the wrists, the muscles around their elbows, shoulders, their lower back and the thigh muscles, the quadriceps and hamstrings which are so important to stretch. I urge them to do a good 15 to 20 minutes' warm-up before they start lifting.
>
> Then they might use a broomstick to go through the routine of warming up their shoulders and going down into the squat position just to go through the movements they are going to do before they start lifting a bar. The bar itself weighs 25 kilograms, so just starting with that is a fair weight.
>
> With gymnasts, it's important for them to work, stretching and flexing the back, shoulders, wrists and elbows, as well as the knees, to properly prepare those muscles.

WEIGHTLIFTING

With any child starting basic weightlifting good learning techniques are very important. Weightlifting can be started at the age of eight or nine, with the right coaching. This means starting with very light weights and using perhaps a junior bar. But, in general, it means just learning the very fluid movements.

Weightlifting involves very precise and quite aesthetic movements. Learning how to do that takes a lot of time and skill. But once a child learns that basic skill, they can build on the weights as they become stronger and bigger. I think one of the great attributes of co-ordinated weightlifting is that even children who have less strength than others of the same age can still learn techniques such as lifting the bar correctly and then build on them as they get stronger.

Learning the proper techniques is very important.

Weightlifting has boomed in the last few years. Twelve years ago a schoolboy competition began in Melbourne with 500 boys. There are now 70 000 in Australia. One of the reasons is an excellent administrative program. Secondly, many of the physical education teachers realise that it's a great sport for all boys and girls in schools to get into because it gives them a knowledge of the use of weights, not to be afraid of how to use them correctly. Weightlifting can be very helpful for any sort of sport.

Clearly, a lot of the 70 000 children won't go on to do weightlifting into adulthood. There are simply not enough facilities. But there is a talent identification program to find the best ten in each division out of those 70 000 throughout Australia and then take them to the Australian Institute of

STRENGTH SPORTS

Sport. The special program there identifies the top 50 in Australia and these boys can be trained further. If we do this every year, we will produce world champions in the next ten years.

In many schools, like De la Salle in Melbourne, every boy in the school enters into the schoolboy clean and jerk program. The other thing which has been introduced is a schools' program which enables boys to compete against each other. We now have an interschool program in Victoria which was introduced in 1987. The three boys who were the inaugural champions were the most unlikely looking boys — two big, lumbering-looking boys and one little fellow. Weightlifting is one of the few sports which allows a differentiation of body size and weight.

The little fellow was only 44 kilograms. No one thought he had any potential for football, basketball, or cricket. He was just too small. But for weightlifting, in his division, he was number one in Victoria and number two in Australia. The two other boys were overweight and too slow for football. They won the heavy divisions in weightlifting.

Weightlifters must have a good ratio of height to body weight.

Weightlifters have to have a good ratio of height to body weight. In other words, they cannot be too tall. They have to have a low centre of gravity to be an extremely successful weightlifter. They must also have tremendous self-discipline and determination.

The major factor for good weightlifting is an excellent technique. Australia has been applauded internationally at a junior level for having the best technique in the world. Our excellent training programs and school programs enable us to teach children how to lift properly and then give them the opportunity to continue developing their skills.

GIRLS AND WEIGHTLIFTING

The success of the schoolboy and schoolgirl clean and jerk competition shows that many girls are also interested in strength sports and in learning how to lift weights correctly, still not as much as boys but the interest is growing.

I personally believe that weightlifting lends itself more to males than females. But certainly girls can successfully learn the proper techniques and lift weights.

STRENGTH SPORTS

Free weights and weight training

There's no doubt that the use of free weights is far superior in any weight training program to using those fantastic-looking machines in gyms. Free weights are now recognised as by far the most effective method of strength training. They put joints, such as the shoulders, elbow and wrist and also the spine, hips and knees, through the full range of movement. This is why so many coaches in football and other sports are now going back to using free weights in sports. I believe weight training has a big part to play in the overall training for a wide range of sports such as football, cricket, basketball, and track and field. The old adage was that runners, including those doing long-distance events, should never lift weights and should just go out there and run. But a back squat, for example, can be done with such power and force that it can build up tremendous strength in the muscles of the legs.

The use of free weights is better than the gym machines.

There is an important difference between power and strength. Strength is just the actual amount of force which can be generated. Power is force times velocity — strength and speed. Weightlifters are very powerful whereas bodybuilders or powerlifters may be very strong. 'Powerlifting' is really the wrong word because powerlifters are not as powerful as Olympic weightlifters. They're strong but their movements are a lot slower. They do the dead lift and the squat whereas weightlifting is also a very dynamic sport.

Weightlifters lift the bar extremely quickly. In fact, few people realise that one of the fastest movements in any sport is the movement of the bar in one snatch from the floor to when it's secured overhead.

Injuries

In terms of injuries, essentially the things to look for are overuse injuries. When children begin to lift more regularly and increase the amount of weights they are lifting, then they're going to get soreness in their wrists, their shoulders and in their knees.

Anterior knee pain is one of the biggest problems.

One of the biggest problem areas is anterior knee pain, that is, pain caused by the inflammation under the kneecap or the patella tendon due to the immense forces being applied through the body when you squat down to lift up the weight and then when holding it overhead.

The shoulders are also vulnerable because of the tremendous rotation in the snatch, and the forces applied to the shoulder joint and the muscles around it can cause muscle strain and inflammation in the capsule joint. The same can happen to the wrist.

STRENGTH SPORTS

Remember, weightlifters hold the bar with the wrist bent back. The amount of pressure applied to the wrist joint can cause irritation. Again, with discomfort but without any really serious injury.

I haven't seen a torn major ligament in the knee in the 12 years I have been involved in weightlifting. I have seen a few meniscal tears and also several muscle ruptures, particularly involving the biceps (upper arm muscles) and quadriceps (the upper thigh and buttocks muscles). These usually involve the older athlete working with heavier weights.

Injuries are not common in the schoolboy and the junior programs. Many people comment to me that surely all weightlifters must have wrecked backs! But the fact is that very few have problems with their lower back apart from having some soreness.

Correct lifting is important to strengthen the muscles.

This again highlights, even with other sports, that correct lifting is very important to strengthen the back muscles and also those around the buttocks region. You can get some muscular strain in the lower back. But serious back injuries are not that common.

Weightlifting is one of the safest sports.

I would rate weightlifting as being one of the safest sports if taught correctly and done sensibly. The program must be well run, children should have a good coach who has probably gone through one of the coaching programs run by the Weightlifting Federation, and there should not be any overcrowding which sometimes happens when there are people trying to lift weights all over the place. People might be dropping bars and suchlike.

There should be good co-ordination and control by a senior person such as a coach or trainer. This is one of the best ways to prevent accidents happening in a gymnasium. Accidents are usually due to neglect and poor management. That's always a problem, as it is with any other sport, such as a high jumper trying to jump too high. Such safeguards again come back to the coach being in control. If you go to the major gyms, there's always close supervision. When you're training for competition, you're gradually pushed to your limit. But it's a limit at which your coach knows you're capable of performing.

STRENGTH SPORTS

Equipment

Good weightlifting boots are not so important when children are just starting off. A good pair of sandshoes is adequate. Then, as they become more involved, it's advisable to get a good pair of weightlifting boots with a strap around the top and also a leather sole and a leather heel to give them a little bit of a lift when they are going through the various movements. The extra support they give is well worth the price.

In weightlifting, you're allowed to have chalk on your hands and, if any blisters appear, they should always be looked after in training. You should always get to them promptly so they don't get infected because this could seriously interfere with the effectiveness of training and competition.

SUMMARY

One of the major issues in weightlifting, and also in gymnastics, is how we can best allow the body to recover from a gruelling training program. The prime treatment of overuse syndromes is prevention or early recognition.

These people train once or twice a day, six days a week, so we have to try to devise a method to help the body to recover from these intense training programs. Sometimes, the training is far more intense than the competition!

We also have to allow the body to recover with massage and attention to vitamins and nutrition, hot baths and saunas and a whole variety of treatments to help the recovery process. I think this is a very important, and often overlooked, aspect of gymnastics and other sports involving intense training.

Ten Golden Rules for Children's Sport

1   ALWAYS REMEMBER THAT CHILDREN ARE NOT LITTLE ADULTS. Never be carried away with enthusiasm. It's always wise to keep a commonsense perspective of your child's physical limits rather than expecting to be able to achieve miracle performances.

2   CHILDREN SHOULD BE PARTICIPATING IN A SPORT BECAUSE THEY WANT TO. They should not be playing because they are being pressured into it by their parents or school. If they are happy about doing a sport, they're going to be a lot less injury-prone.

3   AN ADEQUATE WARM-UP IS ESSENTIAL. It should be appropriate to the type of sport being undertaken. Always seek the advice of your school coach or a qualified sporting instructor if in doubt. Guesswork can be expensive in terms of your son or daughter's welfare. The frustration in being sidelined for weeks or months by a nagging injury could have been prevented. There's also the disruption to family life that such an injury can mean.

4   ALL CHILDREN PLAYING SPORT SHOULD HAVE PROPER EQUIPMENT. Possibly the most important of all equipment is the correct footwear. The proper equipment doesn't necessarily have to be the most costly with a fancy name endorsing it. Good secondhand equipment is always preferable to a new item which is the wrong size, shape or is otherwise unsatisfactory. The importance of you going to the trouble to make sure that all equipment be correctly fitted and matched to the size of the player cannot be overemphasised. For example, tennis racquets should be properly balanced to avoid wrist injuries. They could be better off with a mid-size racquet rather than with an oversize head.

5   CAREFULLY CHECK THE SPORTING VENUE FOR HAZARDS. This applies to a football field and cricket ground for sprinkler heads, fences, seats and other obstructions too close to the boundary, a basketball court for the boundary too close to a wall, an outdoor netball court for broken asphalt, or littered with loose stones, drinks or food litter. In horse riding, the course should always be checked

TEN GOLDEN RULES

out, particularly near jumps so that the rider is aware of possible hazards in case a horse shies at a jump. Knowing what's behind the bushes, trees or around the next bend could mean the difference between salvaging the situation in that split second when you have to make a decision or being thrown and getting back or head injuries.

CONCENTRATION IS A MUST AT ALL TIMES. 6
Always take a few minutes to close your eyes and prepare your mind before any sport. Your mind and your body are partners in the event. Never let anyone play or ride when they are tired, unwell or just feeling out of sorts.

THE FIRST FEW HOURS FOLLOWING THE INJURY 7
ARE VITAL. That is the time to obtain the appropriate treatment to avoid serious complications. Simple commonsense and basic first aid principles, particularly when dealing with soft tissue or muscle injuries, or injuries to a joint, can significantly aid in the recovery from such an injury and also in preventing more significant secondary problems from occurring.

NEVER RETURN TO A SPORT TOO SOON AFTER 8
AN INJURY. Always err on the side of caution, particularly with a head injury. Experience overwhelmingly shows that players are vulnerable to reinjury or will suffer a separate one. This is particularly true in contact sports such as football of all codes.

IF IT'S AN OBVIOUS INJURY, YOU SHOULD APPLY 9
PROPER FIRST AID. The best of all is RICE: rest, ice, compression, elevation. If you are still concerned about how the head, knee or shoulder injury is responding, then seek medical attention from a doctor. Do it promptly. Always accept medical advice about X-rays and being admitted to hospital for observation. Slow, internal bleeding from a head injury can take time to show. If you had a smash in your car, you wouldn't keep driving it. Your body is much more important. Take good care of it. It's the only one you have been issued with. There are no trade-ins!

THE BEST ACCIDENT PREVENTION DEVICE IS 10
YOU. Parents should be involved. Being there can make all the difference between a cut or grazed elbow or a broken arm. It won't take long for the child to get enough confidence to do their own thing. Your son or daughter will also get the reassurance that you really care. So, make the time. It's one of the best investments you can possibly make.

GUIDELINES FOR CHILDREN IN SPORT

Recommendations endorsed by the Australian Sports' Medicine Federation and the American College of Sports Medicine, endorsed by the American Academy of Paediatrics

1 All children should have a musculo-skeletal assessment before embarking upon a training / competition program of long-distance running.

2 Running events primarily designed for adults are not recommended for children prior to physical maturation. Under no circumstances should a full marathon be attempted by children or adolescents.

3 The maximum training distance should be three times the competition distance. Children known to be physically immature for their age should be limited to the maximum recommended distance for the age group below their own.

4 Regular long periods of running on hard surfaces should be avoided.

GUIDELINES

Children should not be encouraged to participate in competitions designed for adults.

5

Weather conditions should be cool.

6

Children should be taught about ingestion of fluids before and during a race or training session.

7

Appropriate clothing should be worn.

8

There is a danger that the time required for training/competition in distance running may preclude a child from enjoying a wide range of social experiences. Study, mixing with other children and developing other skills are important in normal growth and development.

9

Recommended maximum competitive distances.

10

AGE	DISTANCE
Under 12 years	5 kilometres
13–15 years	10 kilometres
15–16 years	½ Marathon
16–18 years	30 kilometres
18 and over	Marathon

Glossary

Achilles-tendinitis: Inflammation of the tendon of the calf muscle at the back of the leg.

Antagonists: Muscles that produce an opposition movement at a joint.

Anterior cruciate ligament: The main internal ligament of the knee.

Anthropometric measurements: A scientific method of classifying people into body types so they can be better matched to sports to enhance performance and minimise injury. For example, tall and agile for basketball. Short and muscular for weightlifting.

Arthrogram: A test involving injecting dye into a joint to assess damage to the surface to give information that an X-ray cannot provide.

Arthroscopy: A simple operation, under anaesthetic, where a small hole is made in the joint in which is inserted a tiny telescope-like instrument with a light source. Doctors can visualise the internal aspects of a joint, be it the knee joint, shoulder, ankle or wrist joint. Through other small holes made in the joint, instruments can be inserted and investigative procedures performed. This avoids the need to make a large incision to open the joint to perform such procedures.

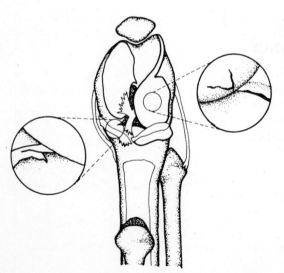

Aseptic avascular necrosis: Death to an area of tissue because of a lack of blood — not due to an infection.

Avascular: Without a blood supply.

Avulsion injury: When either a ligament or a tendon, instead of rupturing when the force is applied, tends to pull off where it's attached to the bone. This is because a tendon or ligament is stronger than the bone, usually in the area where the tendon is attached.

Biceps: A double-bellied flexor muscle in the upper arm.

Biomechanical studies: Studies about the movement of the body, and the forces involved to produce those movements.

Bursa: The sac which is bathing the area with fluid around the common tendon group.

Capital femoral epiphysis: Growth plate head in the thigh bone.

Cartilage: Connective tissue lining part of a joint.

Closed injuries: No open cuts but possible internal bruising or bleeding. A closed head injury can be quite serious.

Collagenous tissues: These include ligaments and capsules. The main purpose of a warm-up is to raise both the general body and the deep muscle temperatures and to stretch the muscles and collagenous tissues to promote greater flexibility.

Collateral ligaments: A ligament supporting either side of a joint. They are not just at the knee, but also at the elbow and other joints.

Concussion: A closed head injury — usually not a subarachnoid nor a subdural which are the big problems. But there is still bruising and damage to some part of the brain tissue which may be serious.

Contusion: A bruise involving slight bleeding into the tissues while the skin remains unbroken.

Corticosteroid: A combination of cortisone and a steroid used as an effective anti-inflammatory treatment.

Cystic lesions: Cyst formation in a tissue.

Developmental lesions: Problems which occur during the growth period.

GLOSSARY

Diathermy: Electrical method of producing heat.

Differential diagnosis: Different causes of a particular problem or symptom. For example, the differential diagnosis of a pain in a joint could be a tumour or a whole range of possibilities.

Divot: An area where there's been an excavation of bone or tissue.

Ectoderm: A lean and tall body type.

Endoderm: A fat and squat body type.

Epiphysis: A growth centre of a bone.

Extensor muscle: One, which on contraction, extends or straightens a part.

Femoral head: The head of the thigh bone.

Femur: The thigh bone.

Fibula: The outer of the two bones forming the lower leg.

Genetic predisposition: An inherited weakness in a person's physical make-up which can mean they are prone to certain injuries.

Glue ears: Condition in which thick fluid collects behind the eardrum in the middle ear. Thus, it's called a middle ear infection because it doesn't drain away into the back of the throat.

Gluteal: Pertaining to the buttocks.

Golfer's elbow: Painful inflammation to the inner aspect of the elbow joint, originally and commonly seen in golfers because of the stress to this area when swinging a golf club. This condition is known as medial epicondylitis.

Growth centres: Embryonic areas in bone from which growth is initiated.

Growth plates: Another name for growth centres.

Haemarthrosis: Bleeding into a joint cavity which is usually rapid and may indicate some significant damage to some internal structure of the joint, such as to a major ligament or a fracture involving the joint or a torn meniscus in a knee joint. Anything which has a good blood supply can bleed into a joint.

Haematoma: A swelling filled with blood. The cause is usually bleeding within the muscle due to damage of the muscle fibres and the small blood vessels within the tissues.

Haemostasis: Stopping bleeding.

Hyperextension: Straightening a joint beyond the normal range.

Hyperthermia: High body temperature.

Hypothermia: Low body temperature.

Iliotibial band: The band of collagenous tissue running on the outer side of the thigh from the hip to the tibia.

Intra-articular fracture: An injury may result to the joint surface cartilage and the maturing bone beneath the surface. Invariably, such a fracture will require an operative procedure for proper re-establishment of a smooth joint surface.

Inversion injury: Common in racquet sports and football, this is the most common ankle sprain in which the foot turns in and under, damaging the outer, or the lateral, ligament.

Isokinetic aspect of muscles: The strength of a muscle through an accommodating force, that is, the greater the pressure applied the greater the resistance.

Isometric muscle strength: The strength of a muscle against an immovable force. For example, applying force through a muscle by leaning against a wall.

Isotonic muscle strength: The strength of a muscle as it's moving a weight against a variable resistance. The resistance becomes greater as it's lifted higher against gravity.

Kinesiology: The study of the motion of joints.

Kohler's syndrome: See *osteochondroses*.

Kyphosis: A rounding deformity of the thoracic spine.

Lateral epicondylitis: The classic description of pain over the outer, or lateral, aspect of the elbow joint. This condition is also called Tennis elbow. While this is common to many sports, it gained its name because it was very common in tennis players caused by the forces generated by their backhand.

GLOSSARY

Medial epicondylitis: See *Golfer's elbow*.

Meniscoplexy: The repair of a torn cartilage by sewing it back. This is only possible if the doctor believes the blood supply is still sufficient for healing.

Meniscus: Cartilage disc in the knee joint.

Mesoderm: A muscular body type.

Myositis ossificans: Calcification of a haematoma — a swelling filled with blood.

Myotatic reflex: A muscle-protective mechanism which is invoked during a stretching manoeuvre.

Navicular bone: Small bone in the foot on the inner, or medial, side.

Neuromuscular co-ordination: The co-ordination of movement involving the nervous and muscular systems.

Open injuries: An open fracture means that the fracture is exposed to the external environment. This means that there's been a laceration through the skin and the wound may be down to the bone. The bone, if broken, is exposed. This used to be called a 'compound' fracture.

Osgood-Schlatter's syndrome: Inflammation and possible separation of the growth plate where the patella tendon attaches to the upper tibia.

Osteochondritis: An inflammation of bone and cartilage.

Osteochondritis dissecans: A defect in the joint-bone cartilage of any synovial joint — knee, wrist, elbow, ankle. An X-ray of the area looks like a divot out of the joint surface.

Osteochondromas: Tumour involving bone and cartilage.

Osteochondroses: An inflammatory process involving both the cartilage and the bone in an area, such as the femoral head (the head of the thigh bone) or the navicular bone of the foot. Other osteochondroses occur in the vertebral bodies of the spine and during adolescence and accounts for postural deformities such as round back (kyphosis).

Overuse syndrome: An injury due to using an area excessively over a long period.

Patella tendon: The tendon of the thigh muscle.

Pathological fractures: A break in a bone which has something wrong with it. For example, a tumour.

Pedicle: A small stalk or stalk-like support, particularly a bony process of the spinal column.

Plantar fascia: The band of tissue which runs across the sole of the foot from the front of the heel bone to the bases of all of the toes. This is a very important ligament because it helps maintain the arches of the foot and prevents the forebones of the foot from spreading out, particularly when taking weight on the foot.

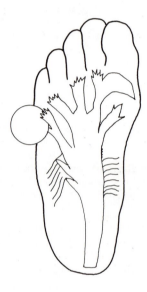

Proprioceptor: One of the body's key sensory receptors responsive to internal stimuli from muscles, joints and tendons.

Quadriceps: Thigh muscles.

RICE: An abbreviation standing for rest, ice, compression and elevation in treating sports injuries.

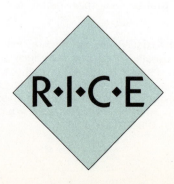

GLOSSARY

Rotator cuff syndrome: Inflammation of a tendon, or a common group of tendons which produce the rotatory movements of the arm at the shoulder joint. This is a common problem with players of racquet sports, basketballers and swimmers.

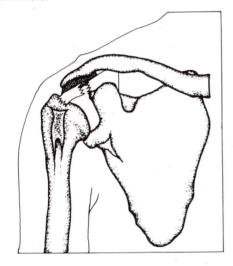

Round back: Kyphosis — a rounding of the spine, usually in the thoracic region. One of the most common causes is Scheuermann's disease in childhood or early adolescence.

Scheuermann's disease: Inflammation of the cartilage lining the vertebral bodies, usually in the thoracic spine.

Sever's disease: A pulling of the insertion of the tendo-Achilles on the back of the heel bone.

Sorbathane: A trademarked artificial shock-absorbent substance used extensively in the inner soles of running shoes.

Subarachnoid haemorrhage: Serious arterial bleeding due to the bursting of an artery resulting in a rapid deterioration in the injured player's condition.

Subdural haemorrhage: Another type of potentially life-threatening brain haemorrhage. A subdural haemorrhage is due to a venous bleed between two layers covering the brain.

Subluxations: The incomplete dislocation of a joint.

Subtalar joint: Just below the ankle joint.

Synovial effusion: Fluid collecting in a joint due to an increased production of the lubricant fluid by the synovium. Overproduction can be caused by a number of factors including loose body in the joint, a tear in the meniscus or irritation of the synovium due to arthritis. This leads to an effusion — a swelling.

Synovial joint: A joint lined by synovium. These are usually the major joints of the body: the shoulder, the elbow, the knee, the ankle. Synovial joints include the small joints in fingers.

Synovium: The inner lining under the capsule beneath the capsule joint.

Tarsal-navicular bone: A key bone in the foot.

Tendinous strength: The strength of a tendon.

Tendo-Achilles: The large tendon of the calf muscle running down the back of the lower leg attaching to the heel bone.

Tendinitis: An inflammation of the tendon usually involving the outer sheath. It can be acute, meaning it can come on very rapidly because of overstress, or it can come on slowly because of overuse. It's commonly seen in children and young adolescents involved in long-distance running or in the upper arms, shoulders or elbows of pitchers or bowlers who have thrown the ball too long or too hard.

Tennis elbow: The classic description of pain over the outer, or lateral, aspect of the elbow joint. See *lateral epicondylitis*.

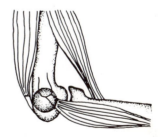

Tenosynovitis: Inflammation affecting a tendon sheath. The condition may be either acute or chronic. Any injury to a tendon sheath may result in tenosynovitis. The symptoms are pain and swelling along the course of the tendon. The usual treatment is RICE: rest, ice, compression and elevation.

Tibia: The major bone in the lower part of the leg between the knee and the ankle.

Trauma: Any injury.

Tympanic membrane: The eardrum.

Vulva: The external area around the vagina.

QUICK-FIND INJURY INDEX

Quick-find Injury Index

A
Achilles tendon 40

B
back pain 65
blisters 42
bone growth, abnormal 26
bruising 61
buttock muscle strain 69

D
dislocation
  finger 50
  shoulder 51

E
ear infections 70
elbow injuries 64, 100
eye infections 69

F
finger dislocation 50
foot injuries 24, 40, 41, 95
fractures 40, 65
function loss 16

H
head injuries 55, 81–83
heel injuries 40, 95
hip injuries 24

I
infection 16

J
joint injuries 16, 17, 25–26, 62
  elbow 64, 100
  finger 50
  knee 39, 52–53, 107, 109
  shoulder 51–52, 63, 97–98, 102
  wrist 97

K
knee injuries 39, 52–53, 107, 109

L
leg injuries 24, 38
limp 24

M
muscle injuries 22, 35, 38, 48, 69

N
neuritis 17

O
overuse syndrome 21, 22

P
pain 16, 17

S
shoulder injuries 51–52, 63, 97–98, 102
spinal injuries 25, 56–57, 65
stress fractures 65
swelling 15, 17

T
tendon injuries 17
  heel 40
  knee 39
tennis elbow 100
thigh injuries 24, 69

W
wounds 15
wrist injuries 97

Index

A
abrasions 46
Achilles tendon 125
  exercises 94
  injury 35, 40, 80, 95, 96, 122
acromioclavicular joint 51–52
age and training 111
alcohol 73
ankle
  injuries 25, 89, 91–94, 105
  pads 89
  sprains 80, 92–93
  straps for surf boards 71, 72
antagonists 122
anterior cruciate ligament 109, 122
anterior knee pain 106, 115
anthropometric measurements 122
anti-inflammatory drugs 17
arena see playing area
arm injuries 35, 62, 75
arthrogram 122
arthroscopy 53, 108, 122
aseptic avascular necrosis 122
aspirin 17
athletics 28–42
avascular 122
avulsion injuries 20, 22, 95, 122

B
back
  injuries 116
  pain 65
badminton 91–102
ball 59
baseball 59–66
basketball 103–109
biceps 35, 122
bicycle riding 75–85
bicycles 75–76
biomechanical studies 122

bleeding in the brain 81–82
blisters 42, 117
Blu-Tac as earplugs 70
BMX bike riding 75–85
body surface area to body mass
  ratio 32
bone
  damage 62
  osteochondroses 23–27
  projections 26
boots
  basketball 109
  bat and ball sports 60
  football 44–45
  netball 105
  skating 89
  skiing 88, 90
boundary lines 61
boxing 87
brain injuries see head injuries
bras 60
breasts 60
breathing difficulties 82
bruising 61
bursa 122
bursitis 37
buttock muscle strain 69

C
calf muscle 35, 40
capital femoral epiphysis 122
cardiovascular fitness 18
cars 77–78
cartilage 20, 108, 122
  injuries 80
  joint surface 25
  meniscus 52, 105, 124
chest injuries 57
chlorinated pools 69
climatic conditions 121
  running 30–31

skiing 90
closed injuries 122
clothing 121
  cycling 77
  skiing 88, 90
cold 73–74
collagenous tissues 122
collapse 82
collar bone fracture 75
collateral ligaments 122
compression of swelling 15
  see also RICE
concussion 83–85, 122
contra coup head injuries 81
contusion 122
corticosteroid 122
cortisone injections 97–98
cricket 59–66
cuts 46
cycling 75–85
cystic lesions 122

D
deformity
  joints 19–20, 62
  spine 25
dehydration 32
developmental lesions 26–27, 122
diathermy 123
differential diagnosis 123
dilation of the pupil 82, 83
dislocations
  finger 50–51
  shoulder 51
distance running 28–42
divot 123
doctors, when to see 16–17
double vision 82
drinks 32, 121

126

INDEX

E

ear infections 69–70
ear-drops 70
earplugs 70, 74
ectoderm 123
elbow
  exercises 94
  injuries 25, 63, 64, 80, 98–100, 111
  pads 80, 86, 90, 109
elevation of limbs 15
  see also RICE
endoderm 123
endurance swimming 72
epicondylitis 123, 124
epiphysis 20, 123
episode trauma 23
equipment 13–15, 118
  selection 12
  football 43, 58
  skiing 88
  weightlifting 117
  see also protective equipment
exercises
  ankles 93
  calf muscle 40–41
  elbow 100
  thigh 49
  football 49
  racquet sports 93
  running 40–41, 42
  swimming 68
  tennis 100
  see also stretching exercises; warming-up
extensor muscle 123
eye
  dilation 82, 83
  drops for 70
  infections 69
  injuries 100–101

F

falls, landing correctly 90
fatigue 11
femoral head 123
femur 19, 23, 123
fibrocystic lesions 26
fibula 39, 123
finger dislocations 50–51
first aid 119
  courses 7
fitness, cardiovascular 18
flags for bicycles 76
fluids 32, 121
foot
  bones 39
  injuries 24, 41, 91–95
  see also Achilles tendon
football 43–58
footwear
  bat and ball sports 60, 66
  racquet sports 91, 101
  weightlifting 117
  see also boots; shoes
forearm fractures 62, 75
fractures 15, 86
  foot 39
  forearm 62, 75
  hip 20
  leg 24, 39
  ribs 57
  spine 65
  tibia 88
free weight training 115
function loss 16

G

genetic predisposition 123
gloves 59
glue ears 69, 123
gluteal 123
goal posts 44
goggles
  for BMX riding 80
  for squash 101
  for swimming 69, 74
golfer's elbow 99, 123
groin injuries 80
groin protectors 59–60
grommets 70
growth centre injuries 19–27, 123
growth plates 123
growth spurts 7–8, 67
gymnastics 110–113

H

haemarthrosis 108, 123
haematoma 123
haemorrhage, brain 81–82
haemostasis 123
hamstring muscle 35, 80
handicapped children 9
handlebar padding 80
head injuries 87
  cycling and skateboarding 75, 81–85, 90
  rugby 55
  surfing 71
headache 82, 84
healing time 17
heel injuries 95, 101
helmets 13, 87
  bat and ball sports 60
  BMX riding and skateboarding 81, 90
  cycling 75, 76–77, 80
  horse riding 85
  skateboarding 80
high jump 31, 42
hip joint
  displacement 20
  pain 23
hockey 59–66
hormonal manipulation 112
horse riding 85–86
hot weather 31
humid weather 31
hyperextension 123
hyperthermia 32, 123
hypothermia 73–74, 123

I

ice 15, 61
  massage 35, 38
  see also RICE
ice skating 89–90
iliotibial band 37–38, 123
infection 16, 46
inflammatory cells 17
intra-articular fracture 20, 123
inversion injury of the foot 92, 123
isokinetic aspect of muscles 123
isometric muscle strength 92, 123
isotonic muscle strength 92, 123

J

jarring injuries 95
joint injuries 16, 20, 50–54, 62, 111
  see also ankle; elbow; finger; knee; shoulder; wrist
joint mouse 25
joint surface cartilage 25
joints, swollen 17

jumper's knee 106
jumping 30, 31, 35, 42

K

kinesiology 123
knee
  bandages 44
  injuries 19, 25, 52–54, 80, 88, 105–9, 111
  pads 86, 89, 90, 105, 109
  pain 24, 115
Kohler's syndrome 24, 124
kyphosis 124

L

landing pits 30–31, 42
lateral epicondylitis 124
leg
  muscle injury 35, 40
  pain 24, 40
  see also knee; thigh
Legg-Perthes syndrome 23–24
lesions
  developmental 26–27
  fibrocystic 26
  rotator cuff 63
ligaments
  feet 41, 95
  joints 74
  knee 19, 52, 53–54, 105, 109
  support for 14
  see also avulsion injuries
limp 20, 23, 95
Little Athletics 28–42
long jump 30, 42
long-distance running 22, 31–32
lungs 57

M

management of participants 10–11
marathons 31
matching children to a sport 9
maturation 8
medial epicondylitis 99, 123
meniscoplexy 124
meniscus 52, 105, 124
mesoderm 124
micro-fractures 24
middle-distance running 35
mismatching children to a sport 9
motivation 11
muscle
  inflammation 97
  injuries 34–37, 47–49
  strain 48, 67–69, 74
  strength tests 92–3
myositis ossificans 124
myotatic reflex 124

N

nausea 55, 82, 84
navicular bone 124
neck injuries 56, 75
  see also spinal injuries
netball 103–109
neuritis 17
neuromuscular co-ordination 124
night cycling 77
non-stretch tape 14, 54
numbness 56
nutrients in healing 17

O

open injuries 124
Osgood-Schlatter's syndrome 24, 107, 124

127

osteochondritis 124
osteochondritis dissecans 25–26, 124
osteochondromas 26, 124
osteochondroses 23–27, 124
overtraining 74
overuse injuries 14, 21–22, 23, 124
   bat and ball sports 66
   gymnastics 110
   running 40
   tennis 97
   weightlifting 115
oxygen in healing 17

P

pads
   bandages 44
   ankle 89
   elbow 80, 86, 90, 109
   knee 86, 89, 90, 105, 109
pain 16, 17
   back 64
   elbow 64
   heel 95
   hip and thigh 23
   knee 106, 107, 108, 115
   leg 23–24
   lower leg 40
   muscle injuries 35
   overuse suyndrome 21
   spinal 56
patella
   femoral joint 80, 111
   tendon 39, 89, 107, 124
pathological fractures 124
pedicle 124
pelvic bone injuries 20, 42
pins and needles 56
plantar fascia 41, 124
playing area 12, 118
   bat and ball sports 61, 66
   BMX 79
   football 43–44, 58
   netball and basketball 104, 109
   running 30, 42
   see also tracks
postural deformities 25
pre-conditioning 12
pre-season training 45, 58
prevention of injury
   ankles 93
   ear infection 70
   eye infections and injuries 69, 101
   athletics 30, 33, 42
   bat and ball games 61
   cycling 78–80, 76–77
   football 43–46, 58
   horse riding 86
   netball and basketball 103–105
   racquet sports 93, 94, 98–99, 101–102
   skating 89
   skiing 88
   water sports 69, 70, 71
   see also protective equipment;
      warming-up
proprioception 14, 124
protective equipment 13
   bat and ball sports 59–60, 66
   bicycles and skateboards 80–81, 90
   football 44
   see also helmets; prevention of injury
pupil dilation 82, 83

Q

quadriceps 124

R

racquet 99, 102
ramps, skateboarding 80
recovery time 17
red eyes 69
referees 43
reflective tape for cycling 77
rest 15
   see also RICE
resumption of sport 18, 39, 102, 119
rib injuries 57
RICE 15–16, 48–49, 124
riding horses 85–86
rotator cuff
   irritation 97
   lesion 63
   syndrome 125
round back 125
rubber pontoons 31
rugby 43–58
rules 12
   modification 9
   bat and ball sports 59, 66
   football 43, 45, 56, 58
running 22, 28–42, 120

S

safety flag for cycling 76
safety vests for water sports 72
sailing 72–73
St John Ambulance first aid courses 7
Scheuermann's disease 25, 125
seat belts in cars 77–78
selecting equipment 12
Sever's disease 95, 125
shinpads 59–60, 60
shoes
   for distance running 32
   netball and basketball 105, 109
   running 42
shoulder
   exercises 94
   injuries 51, 63, 97–98, 102, 111, 115
   muscles 35
skateboard riding 80–85
skating 89–90
skeletal injuries 80
ski stock thumb 89
skiing 88–89, 90
sleepiness 55
slipped epiphyseal 20
snow-skiing 88–89, 90
soccer 43–58
softball 59–66
Sorbathane 125
spinal injuries 25, 42, 55–57, 65, 111
sprains to the ankle 80, 92–93
sprinting 35
squash 91–102
strapping 13, 44
stress, psychological 11, 74
stress fractures 15, 39, 65
stretching exercises
   running 35–36, 38
   swimming 68
stunting of growth 19
subarachnoid haemorrhage 82–83, 125
subdural haemorrhage 83, 125
subluxations 125
subtalar joint 125
support of ligaments 14
surfaces, playing *see* playing area
surfing 71–72
sweat 104
swimming 67–70, 72

swollen joints 17
synovial effusion 108, 125
synovial joint 25, 125
synovium 125

T

tape, non-stretch 14, 54
tarsal-navicular bone 24, 125
tendinous strength 125
tendo-Achilles *see* Achilles tendon
tendon damage 34, 97
   knee 39
   patella 107
   shoulder 63
   see also avulsion injuries; tendonitis
tendonitis 17, 22, 89, 111, 125
tennis 91–102
tennis elbow 98–100, 102, 124, 125
tenosynovitis 125
thigh
   bone 19, 23, 123
   exercises 49, 80
   injuries 35
   muscle strain 69
   pain 23
thumb injuries 89
tibia 125
   fracture 39, 88
   osteochondrosis 24
time of recovery 17
tracks
   BMX 79
   running 30, 42
training, pre-season 45, 58
trauma injuries 14, 125
tricep muscle 35
triple jump 42
tumours 27
tympanic membrane 125

U

ulna collateral ligament 89
umpires 43, 45
unconsciousness 81, 84

V

venue *see* playing area
visor for BMX riding 80
vomiting 55, 82, 84
vulva 80, 125

W

warming-up 10, 118
   bat and ball sports 66
   BMX riding and
      skateboarding 80–81
   gymnastics and weightlifting 113
   netball 109
   racquet sports 94, 98, 102
   running 36, 42
water sports 68, 74
water 32
water sports 67–74
water-skiing 72–73
weather *see* climatic conditions
weightlifting 113–117
wet weather 30
whiplash 56
wounds 46, 104
   ice for 15
wrist
   exercises 94
   injuries 25, 97, 115